PARENTING

The Art and Science of Nurturing

PARENTING
The Art and Science of Nurturing

SHEKHAR SESHADRI
Department of Child and Adolescent Psychiatry
National Institute of Mental Health and
Neuro Sciences (NIMHANS)
Bengaluru, Karnataka

NIRUPAMA RAO
NIRAAMAYAA (a Waldorf-inspired
school for children with special needs)
Mumbai, Maharashtra

BYWORD BOOKS™

First published 2012

10 9 8 7 6 5 4 3 2 1

ISBN 978-81-8193-096-5

Cover design and illustrations: Netra Shyam
Typesetting: Shailesh Mishra, Jacob Thomas

Published by
Byword Books Private Limited
GF-15, Virat Bhavan
Mukherjee Nagar Commercial Complex
Delhi 110009, India; Phone: 011-47038040
email: bywordbooks@gmail.com
website: www.bywordbooks.in

Printed at Manipal Technologies Ltd., Manipal, India

Contents

Introduction

The guys who fear becoming fathers don't understand that fathering is not something perfect men do, but something that perfects the man. The end-product of child-raising is not the child but the parent.

—FRANK PITTMAN, *Man Enough*

The authors hosted 'The Parenting Show' on the Moksha channel of WorldSpace satellite radio in 2005. Each of the 16 episodes featured a different aspect of parenting and a lot of information was written as well as compiled from various sources including libraries and the internet. With so much research, experience and passion for the subject having gone into the making of each episode, it was felt that all this should somehow reach and benefit more people. Hence the idea for this book came into being.

* * *

Awareness, consciousness, prevention—these are some of the words that come to mind when we think about why we wrote this book. Being practitioners in child psychology and psychiatry, we see a number of cases everyday that could have been prevented had the parents been aware of the issue.

If the parents had had an inkling that Aryan's refusal to socialize and make eye contact was a part of his being on the autism spectrum and not due to shyness, they could have initiated an intervention when he was as young as two

If Rhea's parents had been aware that her feelings needed to be recognized and acknowledged rather than judged, they would probably have known that she was depressed before it was too late.

Awareness leads to prevention. The objective of this book is to create awareness among the public so that many issues that have the potential to manifest themselves as complicated problems can be either prevented or at least arrested in a milder form.

Parenting has never been as tough as it is today. Excessive exposure, excessive distractions, excessive independence, excessive materialism, and diminishing spiritual and human values have made parenting tough enough for parents to wake up to the fact that it is all right to seek help.

We hope that with this easy read, parents are able to find some answers to the perplexing questions that come up at various stages in the intriguing journey of raising children, the inevitable consequence of which is growing up along with them!

SHEKHAR SESHADRI
NIRUPAMA RAO

May 2012

Acknowledgements

This book had its genesis in an invitation by Velu Shankar, who asked me whether I could conduct a programme on parenting for the lifestyle and wellness channel, Moksha, on WorldSpace satellite radio. This show did well, with the able assistance of Ashvee and Harish of WorldSpace. It was Nirupama Rao who put together most of the material for the show and, indeed, for this book. Having listened to the concerns of parents for so long, I have always been interested in reaching out to more parents. Of course there were those who came for help, but what of the others? The show on WorldSpace offered me my first opportunity to reach out to larger numbers, even if they were only a part of a niche audience who possessed WorldSpace sets. Many years have gone by since the show was first aired. The publishers, Byword Books, who knew of it, persuaded us to revive the material, and Nirupama diligently reworked the book that you see in its current form. We owe a debt of gratitude to the families that we have served, the institutions where we have trained and those which provide us the space to deliver service, our colleagues whose wisdom and approach have always been inspirational, and our families which remind us of the importance and challenges of unconditional nurturing.

SHEKHAR SESHADRI

* * *

I would like to convey my deepest gratitude to Dr Seshadri for believing that I could be of help to him on this project. I have been enriched as a result of all the interaction and inputs that I have received from him while we were working on this book. It was an honour to work with you, Sir.

I would like to thank Ashvee and everyone on the WorldSpace team that worked on 'The Parenting Show'. It has been of one of the most interesting and cherished experiences of my life.

Thank you, Byword Books, for helping this project see the light of day. Thanks for all the suggestions and editorial help from your team and for giving me a chance to revise a lot of what was written earlier, so that the final product is in alignment with where I am in life today.

I would like to thank all my past and present teachers who have shaped my thinking and are helping me to convert that into willing action. I would also like to thank my parents and all my friends and colleagues who have supported me and contributed their stories and experience to the book. Some names have been changed to protect their privacy.

This book is the compilation of all that was gathered as a result of years of our own clinical and academic experience along with much research on books and articles written on the subject. Unfortunately, technology let me down, and much data that was stored in terms of the sources of information and bibliography were lost when the computer crashed. I have mentioned as many of the sources and authors whose work has contributed to this compilation as I could, but if there is some work that is not referenced, please let me state that we are grateful to all the authors, researchers and scientists who have spent their lifetime working on various subjects connected to children, parents, families and societies.

Most of us learn parenting from our parents, and I would like to thank my mum and dad, Vijaya and Radhakrishna for their sincere, loving and honest efforts in raising my sister and me, and my sister Priya for believing in me.

My dear husband MVN Rao has been a pillar of strength to me over the past 16 years and has helped me evolve as a human being. Travelling together on the sometimes smooth and sometimes rocky boat of parenting has brought us closer to each other and helped us to grow and evolve together.

I am so very grateful to my two daughters Prakruthi and Srishti who continue to teach me unique and valuable lessons for life. They also enable me to be a better professional, helping me to empathize with other parents and to walk the path along with them.

Parenting is not easy, but parenting a child that needs special care is far, far more difficult. I would like to take this opportunity to say 'hats off' to the special parents, especially the mothers who are doing such a fantastic job with their children. Thanks for teaching all the rest of us who take our children for granted and complain about the smallest things, to be patient and to see what is good in our children.

Last but not the least, I want to thank all the children who have touched me at various points in my life, work and practice and have rendered it richer with their mere presence in it. They are my masters and my gurus leading me on my path. This book is dedicated to each and every one of them.

NIRUPAMA RAO

{ Section I }

ISSUES IN EARLY PARENTING

{ Chapter 1 }

Early Stimulation

> *It's not only children who grow. Parents do too. As much as we watch to see what our children do with their lives, they are watching us to see what we do with ours. I can't tell my children to reach for the sun. All I can do is reach for it, myself.*
>
> —JOYCE MAYNARD

How far can you look back? What are the images that come to your mind? A busy household, full of people? Mother's soothing voice? The intoxicating smell of snacks being fried when you came home from school? Being wrapped in the warmth of your grandmother's arms? Listening to her sing songs as old as time itself? Songs about people, songs that told stories, songs that ended with your being tickled all over?

Ah, and stories! Stories of kings and heroes, monsters being slain, going across the seven seas, to a mountain or a deep dark cave. Stories that triggered your imagination and transported you to another world, or your favourite—the stories about the pranks your father played as a child. Don't you remember asking her to tell the same story again and again?

Do you remember colours? Lots of vivid and vibrant colours? The plastic wire baskets that the women of the house used to weave on quiet afternoons, the colourful mobiles (not phones!) hanging from the cradle of your little baby brother?

I am sure we all remember growing up and all our senses being stimulated. These were the building blocks of our personality and of the development of our brain a couple of generations back.

What is meant by early stimulation? Why do we need to know

about it? I am sure our mothers and grandmothers never heard of it, yet we think we are pretty well developed and adjusted.

What is stimulation?

We are all aware that human behaviour is a function of the interaction between heredity and the environment. There are various studies on how heredity and the environment independently affect human behaviour. Studies on stimulation focus on how the environment plays an important role in determining human development and behaviour. A central principle of neural development is that while brain maturation influences children's behaviour, environmental experience also influences neurobiological development.

Stimulation refers to the experiences and activities provided to children that enhance their motor, cognitive (that is, learning), perceptual (sensory), social and emotional development. Stimulation, in other words, is experiential nutrition for the brain.

Why the stress on early stimulation?

At birth, the average infant brain is only one-third the weight of the adult brain. There is a major growth spurt at the age of approximately 4 years, and by the age of 5, the weight of a child's brain is 90% that of the brain of an adult. Much of this increase in size is due to the growth of neurons and their connections.

An important principle of neurobiological development is that synaptic connections strengthen in response to experience. When the different areas of the brain do not receive stimulation, the neural synapses start getting 'pruned'; what is called 'decay through disuse' starts to happen. This loss of synapses can begin as early as the first year of life! Activation of both individual neurons and neural networks in response to stimulation increases the likelihood of the synapses' survival.

Functional evidence reveals that the brain is plastic—almost like raw clay—but only up to a certain age. Young children can even recover from brain damage if their brain areas are activated.

The effects of 'maternal–social' deprivation, institutionalization and hospitalization, and of parental abuse, neglect and indifference upon infant and child development have been well described by many investigators.[1] When an infant is separated and isolated from loving, attentive parents, there is an initial stage of protest, agitation and distressful crying, followed by depression and withdrawn, autism-like behaviour. Profound motor and mental retardation can develop, and movement stereotypes such as rocking are often present.

James Prescott[2] suggests that sensory deprivation during the formative periods of development leads to abnormal development of the deprived system. Depending on the magnitude of deprivation, structural abnormalities of brain cells, i.e. brain damage, can occur. The brain is highly immature at birth and is dependent upon sensory stimulation for normal growth, development and function.

The most important senses that are to be stimulated in the early years, especially up to the age of 7, are the senses of touch, movement and balance, apart from the sense of basic well-being. The stimulation of these senses has a direct impact on brain development.

There are the studies of Dr Mary Neal who constructed a swinging bassinet for premature babies. The premature babies that were given this artificial body-movement stimulation showed accelerated neuromaturation, as reflected in head movements, crawling, grasping and other reflexes. These infants gained weight faster, had less health problems and were discharged earlier from the hospital than premature babies who were not given the stimulation of movement.

In spite of the evident positive effects of auto-moving incubators on the health of premature babies as shown by Dr Neal, such incubators are not in use even in American hospitals. The necessity of movement is mostly overlooked in modern infant care and the newborns are placed on still mattresses.

About 20–30 years back, our lifestyle worked in our favour, providing us with all the stimulation that was required. The traditional Indian village life afforded us with myriad smells, sights, sounds, textures and tastes, along with ample time for free physical play, socializing with our siblings, cousins and friends, and learning to help, share and chip in with the household chores.

Why is this particularly relevant now?

Let us look at today's average urban middle- and upper-middle class child whose parents are both employed. Do you think these children are getting the same amount of stimulation as we did? Where are the grandmothers? Where are the siblings? *Where are the mothers?* Today's mothers are busy at work. They are educated and career-oriented. Their time is now divided between work and family.

With the disintegration of the joint family, grandmothers have given way to live-in maids and babysitters, most of who come from impoverished backgrounds and families. What kind of stimulation can they be expected to provide? Young children looked after by babysitters are the worst sufferers of the lot. They are all alone for most part of the day, with only the television for company.

This is also the age of instant coffee and instant dinners. Today's parents want instant prodigies and want to start their children off early. Children are enrolled in various programmes to get trained in dance, music and mathematics. These structured programmes are accepting children at very young ages. Pre-schools are sprouting in every street, claiming to increase the tots' brain power—all stressing on brain development. Aggressive marketing is leading desperate and gullible parents to believe that children are all brains and nothing else. Nothing can be further from the truth.

Research indicates that along with the brain, a child's body also develops at a tremendous pace in the first seven years. In fact, babies triple their birth weight in the first year. A keen observer would notice that young children live in their limbs: constantly moving and playing. Early emphasis on academics deprives children of this natural way of learning, by experiencing the world.

CASE STUDY

The child was two years old. She was her parents' only child. Her father was posted in a foreign country and her mother, hitherto used to all the domestic help in India, had to manage the household work all by herself. They had no friends or neighbours in that alien country. The child's only companion was the television set. Her mother found the television set a blessing as she could finish all her chores while the TV kept the child engaged. Sometimes she would watch TV for five hours at a stretch. Her mother confessed one day, after three years, that she was unaware that she should talk to or play with her child. Neither her mother, nor her mother-in-law had told her to do so.

The child, who had not been stimulated (talked to, played with, been exposed to various sensory experiences) as all young children are supposed to be, was later diagnosed with expressive speech delay, attention deficit and also the risk of being on the autism spectrum.

The early years need to be spent on allowing children to play naturally with the simplest of toys, with nature, working with their hands and moving with their whole being. The early years are not for confining children into cramped pre-schools, unrealistically expecting them to sit still, to not fidget, to not move, laugh, share, talk or play. Academic lessons can always be learnt, but once children cross the critical age, it is not possible to teach them to balance, to move, to learn fine motor movements, to grip, to listen and to communicate clearly.

Early stimulation is necessary; it needs to involve all the senses, including balance and movement. Children need to sense the world with all their being. It is irrelevant to try to make them learn through CD-ROMs and worksheets at an early age. The more they sense the world, the more sense they can make of the world they live in.

What happens if the child does not get enough stimulation?

Since it is unethical to intentionally deprive children for research purposes, the information we have comes from animals and a few naturally occurring unfortunate cases of deprivation in humans.

The Wild Boy of Aveyron

One of the best authenticated cases is that of the Wild Boy of Aveyron.[3] Discovered at the age of about 12, digging in a garden in the Aveyron district of France in 1800, the wild boy was mute, naked and seemingly retarded. It was learnt that he had been roaming the hills on his own for at least two years, living on handouts from obliging farmers and whatever he could steal. The boy was turned over to a determined doctor named Jean Itard, who taught him to dress himself and perform simple chores. However, he never learned to speak more than a couple of words.

Feral (animal-like) children have long fascinated scientists. Apart from the sheer pathos of their stories, they raise some basic issues: How do we become human? If we fail to learn critical skills as children, is it impossible to do so later? Most feral children are severely stunted and remain so all their lives, suggesting that early human contact is essential to normal development.

A 1970 California case suggests that the deprivation theory is valid. 'Genie',[4] a more-or-less normal two-year-old, was locked up by her demented father for 11 years. This reduced her to a state of whimpering imbecility. Despite the training she was given later, her language development never exceeded that of a five-year-old. Being a wild child may conjure up some Tarzan-like visions, but the reality is unspeakably cruel.

More stories

'Rock A Bye Baby',[5] a Time-Life documentary, shows how retardation can be reversed in a retarded institutionalized infant of six months of age if he is provided with a loving substitute mother with whom he forms an intense 'one-to-one' relationship. The longer the period of deprivation and the later a loving mother-substitute is provided in such cases, the lower is the level of recovery from the damage.

In the local Montessori and pre-schools closer home, in Bengaluru, it was found that the children about three years of age who were the quietest in their schools in terms of both language and socialization, had, over a period of more than a year, been spending the entire day with a babysitter, in addition to watching television for long hours. The chief complaints mentioned were those of expressive speech delay and lack of socialization.

At-risk babies

The danger of brain damage due to environmental and sensory deprivation is greater for babies who are 'at risk'. Babies falling in the following categories are at risk:

- Babies with a family history of autism, psychotic illnesses such as suicide, depression and schizophrenia, learning disabilities, epilepsy, mental retardation, and so on.
- A baby is at risk if his mother had a traumatic pregnancy in terms of some illness which may have required intensive medication; if she suffered from rubella, poisoning, exposure to X-rays, injury, or emotional upheavals such as stress and depression during pregnancy; or if she smoked, consumed alcohol or took drugs during pregnancy.
- A baby who suffered trauma during birth is at risk. This would include premature delivery, underweight, delayed birth-cry causing asphyxiation, head injury and traumatic birth process.
- A baby is at risk if he suffers sensory deprivation caused by abandonment by the mother either due to post-partum depression or unwanted pregnancy.

- A baby is at risk if post-natally, i.e. after birth, he develops severe illnesses such as meningitis or high fever, due to which he gets seizures or head injury, is malnourished, or suffers severe sensory deprivation.

Children who fall into any of these categories may be more easily affected by environmental deprivation or understimulation.

If you are aware that a baby is at risk, please note that good stimulation is all the more necessary for this child if he is to develop to his fullest potential.

How do we stimulate our children?

Stimulation need not mean buying expensive toys. All it takes is some tender, loving care and your precious time. Use material available at home—children love playing with discarded boxes, newspaper, kitchen utensils, and water, sand and chocolate wrappers. You can even make dolls out of wrappers and keep your child entertained for hours doing puppet shows! Of course something indispensible is your patience and ability to be present.

Make sure your child gets all types of stimulation. Giving your child stimulation should be woven into your daily routine. The child should be given stimulation for all the senses—expose him to different types of smells, sights, sounds, textures, movements and tastes. The child also needs to get language, social and emotional stimulation. Remember that the games which are to be played vary according to age, progress in behaviour, needs and interest. The important thing is to have fun. If you're having fun, so will your child.

- Songs, verses, finger games, rhymes, naming of plants and animals as well as storytelling should become a habit for parents.
- Take time to attentively listen to your child.
- Touch and massage your child often.
- Play with your child as frequently as you can.

- Expose your child to different sights, sounds and surroundings.
- Ask the child to join you in household work, such as cleaning and gardening.
- If your child falls, do not fret over him and pick him up the second he falls down. Let him get up on his own. He will be fine.
- Allow your child to explore and discover things on his own while providing a danger-free environment and plenty of safe, natural, appropriate toys—even unfinished toys such as boxes, wooden blocks, pieces of a log, shells, stones, etc.
- Remember, your child learns by imitating you. Model behaviour that you want your child to learn. Would you prefer that your child sees you engrossed talking over your phone and imitates that, or would you rather he/she imitates you while you are actively working with your hands?
- Sing and play music to your child even before birth. Generally, music that has a constant rhythm is the best. It is better for you to sing in your own voice.
- To encourage active imagination start telling stories to your child at a young age.
- Make effective use of your travel time together. Talk about things, places and people you see on the way.

> Children are God's gift to us, and how we raise them is our gift to the world. In losing ourselves to the rat race, and our preoccupation with competition and acquiring status symbols, let us not forget to enjoy these gifts. Children are a great source of joy, fun, laughter and relaxation. They have a right to optimum and wholesome development. Let us not deny them these rights. Let us enjoy our children and let us help them to enjoy their lives.

- Allow him to be strong and independent. Allow your child to falter and make mistakes while learning something new. Do not offer to do things for him and make him depend on you for everything.

We need to take care not to over-stimulate our children. (This is discussed in greater detail in a subsequent chapter.) Children today are in danger of being over-stimulated by excessive sensory assault (sounds, visuals) by way of television, video games, car stereos, malls, arcade games, etc. Children need to have calm, peaceful, natural surroundings to grow up in a healthy, balanced way.

{ Chapter 2 }

Developmental Issues—Early Detection and Intervention

Your living is determined not so much by what life brings to you as by the attitude you bring to life; not so much by what happens to you as by the way your mind looks at what happens.

—KAHLIL GIBRAN

The first seven years of life are the most important, when the child's brain and body are mouldable like clay. The maximum development takes place in this phase as compared to any other stage in life. Not all children develop in the same way or at the same pace.

Nevertheless, it is vital to closely monitor the child's development at this stage to ensure that he is developing optimally. It is often not enough to look at only the milestones of development, such as sitting, crawling, standing and walking. For instance, in the case of autism, the common milestones mentioned above could develop at the normal stages, but other equally important signs are easily missed out. Knowledge of child development and awareness of the signs of developmental delay give parents and children an opportunity to enjoy the golden period of development and to seek assessment and intervention where required.

The signs are subtle and can easily be missed even by paediatricians if they are not sensitized. Paediatricians and pre-school teachers are in the best position to observe children in this age closely enough to be able to detect differences in growth patterns.

In this chapter, we attempt to increase awareness among the public so that they can look out for early signs or red flags for the detection of developmental delays. This is not meant to serve as an encouragement to label the children in any way. We all have one or the other of these symptoms. These symptoms should not be considered in isolation. Conditions such as autism, attention deficit hyperactivity disorder (ADHD) and learning disabilities (one of which is dyslexia) are syndromes; i.e. two or more symptoms appear together. The only reason for detection is to start suitable intervention early enough so that every child has an opportunity to develop as close to what is defined as normal (which is changing everyday!) as possible.

There has been an alarming increase in the incidence of developmental issues in early childhood. These include autism, hyperactivity, learning disabilities and sensory processing disorders. Children with these problems, unlike mental retardation, can show a marked improvement if they are diagnosed early and intervention is immediate. Young parents, particularly, should be alert and look out for these symptoms, either in their own children or in any other children whom they meet, and immediately seek assessment. It is best that parents recognize these symptoms on their own; for, often when it is pointed out by a third person, there are chances of their going into denial and losing precious time.

Let us begin by looking at one of the most frequently diagnosed syndromes today.

Autism

Autism is a neuro-biological disorder, first documented by Leo Kanner in 1943. It is one part of the autistic spectrum disorders (ASDs), which includes pervasive developmental disorder (PDD), autism, Asperger syndrome, semantic pragmatic language disorder, or atypical autism; even ADHD.

The basic features of ASD are:

- Impairment in social development
- Impairment in language development and communication
- Restricted and repetitive activities.

The associated symptoms are lack of pretend-play and eye contact, not responding when called and disturbances in the perceptual functioning. It is often mistakenly assumed that three-quarters of all persons with autism are mentally retarded because autism prevents these persons from expressing themselves. Many of them possess average to extremely high levels of intelligence and also savant skills, such as a photographic memory. Such children have shown the ability to memorize an entire telephone directory, as portrayed beautifully by Dustin Hoffman in the film *Rainman*. The physical development and other milestones are normal.

IQ tests are often unable to correctly gauge the actual intellectual functioning of these individuals because such individuals are unable to properly express, communicate or follow commands or instructions. Their actual intellectual abilities go undetected and retardation is assumed. Although they are intellectually endowed, they are unable to apply it in real life and in social situations. This is owing to their lack of social skills and inability to connect to other people. We know much more about autism and ASD today thanks to digital technology, which has enabled such persons to key-in their thoughts and feelings as an alternative to writing (which is very challenging for them due to their poor motor skills). However, parents should not make the mistake of giving keyboards, iPads and other gadgets to such children too early in their eagerness to help children communicate when they should be developing their physical, motor and sensorial skills.

There has been an almost epidemic increase in the incidence of autism and other pervasive developmental disorders in the past few years. Ten years ago, the incidence was 1 in 10,000 and is now an alarming 1 in 125. Autism occurs four to five times more in boys than in girls.

Causes

There is much speculation about the causes of autism and many theories have been advanced to establish various causes. The causes postulated include various types of pre-, peri- and postnatal insult and injury to the foetus and the baby, illnesses or injury during infancy and abnormality on an electroencephalogram (EEG). Recently, the disorder is being associated with immunological causes such as measles–mumps–rubella (MMR) vaccine and food allergies.

Studies have shown that there is a difference in the brain structure of autistic and non-autistic individuals. Genetic studies have shown that there is a higher incidence of autism in the twins and siblings of autistic people. Scientists believe that autism is the outcome of the interaction of genes and environmental offenders, including toxins in the air, vaccines, processed food, electromagnetic radiation and excessive use of antibiotics/paracetamol. Prolonged exposure to television in the case of children below three years of age and poor parental communication skills may or may not be causes of autism, but could make things worse for children with an inborn genetic predisposition. A correlation has been found between autism and a family history of psychiatric illnesses.

Early signs

In about 30% of children who develop autism, the symptoms are evident from the beginning, while others seem to develop normally until a particular age (about 1–3 years of age) and then start losing skills (speech and social skills) that they had already developed. The early signs start showing as early as 1 to 1½ years of age. Unfortunately, these signs are missed both by parents and paediatricians due to lack of awareness. The child is mistaken to be just a shy child with speech delay, which is common among male children, and it is believed that he will outgrow it.

Research has shown that the earlier the child is diagnosed and intervention started, the better is the prognosis. One must remember that there is no cure for autism as it is not a disease but a developmental condition. The prognosis depends on the child's level of intelligence and the kind of care and intervention he receives.

CASE STUDY

Giving birth to a child is the culmination of a couple's dreams. Parents pin all their hopes and desires on their child. They dream of a future when their child will make them proud with his/her accomplishments. This young doctor couple was no different. They were very proud of their child, a three-year-old boy who expressed intelligence in everything he did. He knew the names of all the makes of cars plying on the roads. What they were not aware of was that his teachers felt that he was different from the others. He would play alone, that too, with the same toy and in the same manner every day. If he wanted to go out, he would not say so, but he would take the teacher by her hand and place her hand on the handle. He would sing jingles and name cars, but not speak. He would not play with the other children. He would not respond when the teacher called him. He was afraid of the swings and would go out to play after all the children came back in. He was referred for assessment.

When parents were told that the boy was showing features of autism, they went ballistic. They could not accept it in spite of the fact that the mother, being a doctor herself, had had doubts and been on the internet to find out why their son was different from other children. With no two children showing the same signs, the online test that the mother took turned out to be negative for autism; so she was relieved. The parents could not bear that their suspicions could be true after all and they went into a mode of complete denial. They were worried about the label and did not start interventions in the areas in which the child was lagging behind his peers. This was because even their paediatrician assured them that since he was a boy, he would start speaking late and that since his eye contact was good, they should not worry. What the child specialist and the parents missed were the subtle signs, such as the failure to imitate, point or pretend-play—important indications of autism that are easily missed.

Intervention in the form of special education, speech therapy and occupational therapy, special diets, animal-assisted therapies and certain lifestyle changes will help the child in various areas of impairment. Appropriate intervention will also help to mainstream the child into society in terms of education and employment.

At-risk babies

Parents of children with the following risk factors need to keep a watch on whether the child is progressing normally:

- A family history of psychiatric illnesses, epilepsy, mental retardation, learning difficulties, suicide, depression, etc.
- Illness, injury, substance abuse or emotional trauma during pregnancy
- Difficult, prolonged labour, birth trauma, delayed birth cry, premature delivery, underweight baby
- Illness right after birth or during infancy, such as meningitis, high fever leading to seizures, and head injury
- Prolonged diarrhoea or constipation during infancy, caused by allergy to milk and wheat products (it is speculated that this causes a leaky gut which, in turn, affects the brain and causes symptoms of autism)
- Chronic ear infections and otitis media requiring the insertion of grommets.

Such children run the risk of developing disorders such as autistic spectrum disorder, learning disability, mental retardation or disorders of expressive and receptive language.

Parents who are aware that their child has any of these risk factors need to be alert in monitoring the child's growth and development and should get him periodically assessed for development. The earlier the child is diagnosed, the better will be the prognosis, as the brain is plastic until the age of 5 years and can be moulded to a large extent.

Developmental markers[6]

It is important to realize that no two children grow at the same rate. At the ages noted for different activities, the child should be observed for some time. The child may develop more slowly in certain areas than other children of the same age while his other activities may be ahead of other children.

These markers are not rigid or fixed. Each child is a unique individual. She* follows her own individual pattern of growth. There are early developers and late developers. These are individual patterns, and as any child specialist will tell you, not a cause for concern. However, a check-up by a paediatrician is needed to rule out any medical complication and put the parents at ease.

At 12 months

- Uses a few gestures, one after another, to get needs met, such as giving, showing, reaching, waving and pointing
- Plays peek-a-boo, patty cake or other social games
- Makes sounds such as '*ma*', '*ba*', '*na*', '*da*' and '*ga*'
- Turns to the person speaking when her name is called.

At 15 months

- Exchanges with you many back-and-forth smiles, sounds and gestures in a row
- Uses pointing or other 'showing' gestures to draw attention to something of interest
- Uses various sounds to get needs met and draw attention to something of interest
- Uses and understands at least three words, such as '*mama*', '*dada*', 'bottle' and 'bye-bye'.

* 'She' is used to denote both boy and girl.

At 18 months

- Uses several gestures with words to get needs met, such as pointing or taking you by the hand and saying, 'want milk'
- Uses at least four different consonants in babbling or words, such as m, n, p, b, t, and d
- Uses and understands at least 10 words
- Shows that she knows the names of familiar people or body parts by pointing to or looking at them when they are named
- Engages in simple pretend-play, such as feeding a doll or stuffed animal, and attracts your attention by looking up at you.

At 24 months

- Engages in pretend-play with you with more than one action, such as feeding the doll and then putting it to sleep
- Uses and understands at least 50 words
- Uses at least two words together (without imitating or repeating) and in a way that makes sense, such as 'want milk'
- Enjoys being with children of the same age and shows an interest in playing with them, perhaps giving a toy to another child
- Looks for familiar objects that are out of sight when asked.

At 36 months

- Enjoys pretending to play different characters with you or talking on behalf of dolls or action figures
- Enjoys playing with children of the same age, perhaps showing and telling another child about a favourite toy
- Uses thoughts and actions together in speech and in play in a way that makes sense, such as 'sleepy, go take nap' and 'baby hungry, feed bottle'
- Answers 'what', 'where' and 'who' questions easily
- Talks about interests and feelings about the past and the future.

Early indicators of developmental problems

We have not included early indicators of mental retardation and cerebral palsy here as most forms of mental retardation have obvious signs and are identified easily. The diagnosis of autism and learning disability is missed out more often since the signs are subtle. The chances of early detection are much lower for autism and learning disability. In India, about 20,000 cases of autism are diagnosed every year.

Autism

A doctor should evaluate a child for autism if she displays any two of the following after her first birthday:

- Does not gesture (point, wave, etc.)
- Does not respond to her name when called
- Does not show an interest in other children
- Does not bring objects to show to an adult
- Does not look at a toy pointed out across the room
- Does not imitate facial expressions or actions
- Makes stereotypical movements of hands, fingers (flapping)
- Bites her own hands or inflicts some other form of self-injury
- Does not babble or coo by 12 months of age
- Does not say single words by 16 months of age
- Does not say two-word phrases on her own (rather than just repeating what someone says to her) by 24 months of age
- Has any loss of any language or social skill at any age.

Not all children display all the symptoms. No two children with autism are the same. Hence, therapy programmes for autistic children have to be tailor-made according to their needs and strengths. These children are very uneven in their abilities. They may be very good at remembering routes or names, but cannot say which number comes first. If there is a doubt that the child is showing any of the symptoms mentioned earlier, the parents need to take her to a specialist (paediatric neurologist, psychiatrist, psychologist) or an institution such as the National Institute of Mental Health and Neuro Sciences (NIMHANS), any major hospital in that city, the Spastic Society, etc. for further assessment and diagnosis. Parents should not be afraid of labelling or diagnosis because diagnosis often helps them seek the right kind of help for the child. Online resources are available for parents seeking help.

Autism and issues with communication

Children with developmental delay often develop speech late. Parents frequently make the mistake of not talking to them as they do not respond. Some children who are likely to develop speech later may suffer because of this as their vocabulary does not develop and they have not heard enough language to be able to use it in speech. However, their intelligence and receptive language level may be excellent.

Very often, autistic children are non-verbal. It is just that they may not want to or may not have the will to speak, but they may have the ability to communicate and to even write books. Temple Grandin (USA) and Tito and Krishna of India, people with autism, have become famous for their ability to write and provide a window to their world through their writings and poems.

The parents should focus on teaching the child to 'communicate' and not lay too much stress on speech per se as this puts too much pressure on the child and reduces her confidence and self-esteem. More emphasis needs to be laid on what the child can do rather than on what she cannot.

Learning disability

A child should be evaluated for learning disability if he or she displays any two or more of the following symptoms:

- Late talking, compared to other children
- Difficulty with pronunciation
- Slow growth of vocabulary—the child is often unable to find the right word
- Difficulty in rhyming words
- Trouble learning numbers, the alphabet, days of the week
- Extreme restlessness and getting easily distracted
- Trouble interacting with peers
- Persistent difficulties in getting dressed efficiently and putting shoes on the correct feet
- Poor ability to follow directions or routines
- Excessive tripping, bumping into things and falling over
- Difficulty with catching, kicking or throwing a ball; with hopping and/or skipping
- Difficulty with clapping a simple rhythm.

Early intervention

Regardless of whether or not the child is showing the symptoms listed above, the parents of children who are 'at risk' (and even of those who are not) need to stimulate their children right from birth in all the areas of development, including motor, sensory, language, cognitive and social, within the first five years. This will help children reach their optimum growth potential given their birth and family history. (*See also* Chapter 1: Early stimulation)

The message of autism

The outbreak of autism, ADHD, allergies, asthma and other new-age conditions is prompting many of us to ponder over certain questions, such as why they are on the rise. Is there a message for all of us in this and some lessons for us to learn?

Many parents, especially the mothers of children with autism, feel guilty and responsible for the way their children are. This is neither fair, nor necessary. In fact, all of us are guilty and responsible for the increase in the incidence of autism and other conditions such as ADHD, learning disability, asthma and allergies (even cancer). If we look at what these children are allergic to (everything that is synthetic and toxic), a picture begins to emerge. It becomes clearer when we see how the world has changed over the years. If we ask ourselves why there is an increase in the incidence of these conditions, we will begin to understand that it is because we are moving away from all that is natural, from real human contact and more towards technology. We are making this world too toxic a place for our children to come into—physically, mentally and spiritually.

All children, especially those on the spectrum, are *pure* beings who are not capable of negative thoughts. They are sensitive and vulnerable. They thrive in a pure, calm, non-toxic environment, which is today not available to them. Let us stop and think about how we grew up, how we played, what we ate, the number of loving people we were surrounded by, and how our childhood was—free and without pressure; and then let us look at how children are growing up today. People say that we need to keep up with the times, but then we have to pay a price for it. Our children have to pay a price for it.

We think we need to bring a change in their behaviour, but what we need to realize is that first we need to change. We need to become more conscious and provide all young children with an atmosphere that is calm, quiet, peaceful, clean and pure. Not surprisingly, this is what our Mother Earth needs too. She is trying to talk to us through these children! We must stop and question the choices we are making... not just the parents of children with autism, but all of us.

If we listen intently, we will understand that these children are trying to convey these messages for all humanity through their condition:

- *Be in touch with Mother Nature.* Human beings are products of nature. We cannot afford to forget that. When we are in harmony with nature, we are in balance and healthy. Children calm down in quiet natural places as they are at one with nature. They have not fully separated from it. They tell us to be aware of and follow the repetitive and predictable rhythms of nature. Being random and whimsical makes them feel insecure. They tell us to make nature a part and parcel of our life, in terms of what we eat, what we drink and how we entertain ourselves.

- *Early stimulation is not limited to stimulation of the brain.* A human being has many aspects besides the brain. In the early years, we need to develop a child's senses, physical body, emotions and will. Parents are falling into the trap of providing early brain stimulation at the cost of neglecting other aspects that we got as children. Many children with autism are intellectually gifted. Their weakness lies in their 'will' to do. We need to develop this by providing a proper diet and healthy routines, and emphasizing the senses of touch, movement, balance and natural rhythms.
- *Children are affected by and learn from 'who we are' and not 'what we say or do'.* Our state of being as a parent or a teacher has a direct bearing on their well-being. If we are well, so are they.
- *Children with the conditions we have talked about are very sensitive to their environments.* Many parents of children with autism will vouch for the fact that their children are calmer in positive, non-judgemental environments. We need to refrain from being judgemental about ourselves and others; nobody is perfect.
- We should not dwell in the past or worry (plan objectively, but not worry) about the future. Instead, we should enjoy the present.
- Technology and wealth should be used for the betterment of life and society, and on no account should we become slaves to them.
- Slow down! Calm down!

When parents are able to follow these guidelines, we find that their children are much calmer and begin to show improvement in many areas of development.

We need to become conscious of our choices and make suitable

What can parents do when they find that their child is sensitive (touchy, easily upset, hurt or provoked) or has problems with attention? The following will help the child become more grounded, calm and balanced:

- Stick to natural, home-made food. Avoid sugars, artificial flavours, additives, preservatives and colours.
- Exposure to electronic devices, such as television, mobiles and microwave ovens should be minimized as they release electromagnetic radiation, which could be harmful for children.
- Follow regular rhythms, i.e. there should be a predictable order or sequence in which things are done every day. It is good to have daily, weekly, monthly and yearly rhythms. Get children acquainted with festivals and celebrations.
- Expose children to nature. Go to natural places during weekends and holidays.
- Let the children do a lot of work with their hands and even do real work at home with their hands. Let them touch different kinds of natural textures and even walk on different textures.
- Massage their feet with cream or any warm oil using gentle circular movements before they go to sleep every night. After massaging each foot, make the child wear cotton socks.
- Keep the child warm. It is good to make him wear a vest inside his shirt. Warmth in sensation and warmth in our approach—both are required.
- Make sure children are not over-stimulated. There should not be an overdose for any of the senses. They need to be in a calm, quiet atmosphere. There is no need to have the television or music playing all the time.

and healthy changes in our lives to enable our children to cope with the world. We need to look at the deeper causes of the problems our children are facing and deal with those, such as food intolerance and lack of healthy rhythms and healthy emotional environments, rather than try to 'cure' or 'treat' the symptoms.

We need to get together and work towards *prevention*. This is the time to join hands and do what our children want us to do—create a better, cleaner world and develop healthy lifestyles. Together, we can prevent and reduce the incidence of autism, ADHD, asthma, allergies, obesity, malnutrition and childhood heart diseases, and increase the 'well-being' quotient of the world.

{ Section II }

PARENTING STYLES

{ Chapter 3 }

Discipline and Child Behaviour

Don't worry that children never listen to you; worry that they are always watching you.

—ROBERT FULGHUM

Vishal would come home from school every day, put away his shoes, socks, school bag and lunch bag; wash up, change, eat or drink what his mother had given him; finish off his homework; and then go to play. What do you think when you hear something like this? 'Wow! What a *disciplined* child Vishal is! His mother must be such a good *disciplinarian*!'

There is this other boy, Sonny, who flings his shoes anywhere he wants, throws his bags where he pleases, and starts watching television without even changing. We think of him as an *undisciplined* child. He will need a lot of '*disciplining*'. That sounds like a scary word!

This brings to mind the character of the school principal in the film 'Matilda', Stern. She is unsmiling and whip-wielding, with a menacing look. Or even take the example of an army chief or a PT teacher who 'disciplines' the soldiers or students who make the slightest mistake by commanding them to run around the ground five times! In this illustration, discipline is equated with punishment or 'corporal punishment', as it is 'unpopularly' referred to.

What is disciplining really about?

Is this what discipline is all about? Terrorizing children into doing what adults think they should be doing? Using sheer force to teach the value of discipline? Hitting, spanking, punishing and using other negative methods?

What is the guarantee that the child will do what you want him to do in your absence? There is no guarantee, as what needs to be taught is not internalized. *Internalization* does not take place when the child does not realize *why* something should be done.

For example, there are traffic signals and people are expected to follow traffic rules. There are two types of people. One type follows the rules because the policeman is standing there and if he does not follow the rule, he can be fined. It is most likely that he will not follow the rule when the policeman is not there. This is because he has not internalized or properly understood why these rules are made. He does not completely fathom the danger that he causes not only to himself but also to others by not following safety rules.

The second type will stop at a red light whether or not the policeman is present, because he does not believe in taking risks or chances that could put him or others in danger. This man has internalized the reason for having these rules.

Real discipline has nothing to do with shouting, scolding or spanking. Discipline really means to set clear rules for our children, to let them know their limits and consequences, and to consistently follow through with that. Firm discipline works when:

- We use every opportunity we have to express how much we enjoy being with our children and demonstrate our love for them.
- We do not get all emotional and lose control over ourselves. Children are more likely to listen to us when we are in control. Forget yelling, we do not even have to raise our voices! Sometimes even a look is enough.
- We set examples by doing what we want our children to do.

When we do the above, we can expect children to internalize rules. Children feel secure when they know that their parents are stronger than them. (Keen parents can refer to the blog by Carrie, 'The Parenting Passageway' for beautiful ideas on peaceful parenting.)

Yes, parenting can be peaceful, fun and joyous when one believes that it is possible.

Types of parenting

During the early 1960s, psychologist Diana Baumrind conducted a study on more than 100 children of pre-school age.[7] She identified four important dimensions of parenting. Each of these has a bearing on the child's future adjustment:

- Disciplinary strategies
- Warmth and nurturance
- Communication styles
- Expectations of maturity and control

On the basis of these dimensions, Baumrind suggested that the majority of parents display one of three different parenting styles.

Authoritarian parents are controlling, demanding, threatening and punishing. They believe their children should obey them because

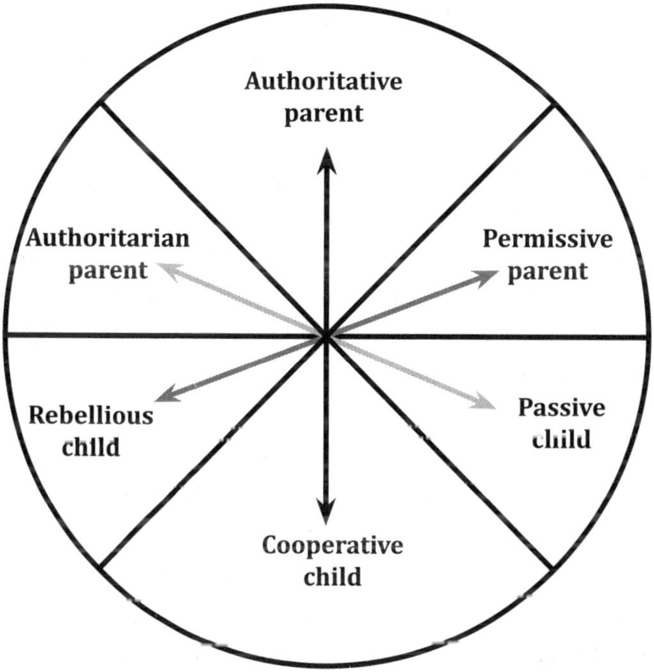

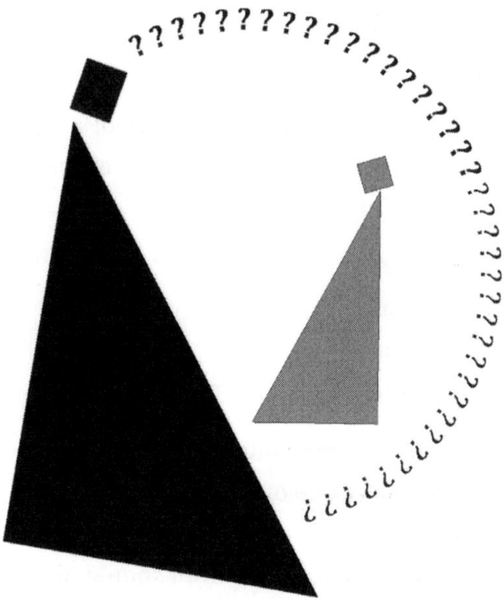

'they say so'. They also believe that 'parents are always right'. They never bother to explain the rules or explain what they want the children to do. This kind of parenting could lead to moodiness, irritability or aggressiveness in the child, or put the child at risk of developing behavioural disorders such as lying, conduct disorders and oppositional defiance disorders.

Authoritative parents, on the other hand, are caring and emotionally available, set appropriate limits, maintain structure and consistency, explain the reasons for rules, and have reasonable expectations from their children and from themselves. This kind of parenting style leads children to be independent, have strong social skills and be confident about themselves.

Permissive parents are loving, emotionally available, accepting and encouraging, and set few limits. Although they sound almost ideal, there is a problem, which is that they do not set appropriate limits. These parents are taken advantage of. The children are spoilt and hence, turn out to be unhappy. They are impulsive and have behavioural problems due to lack of structure and lack of

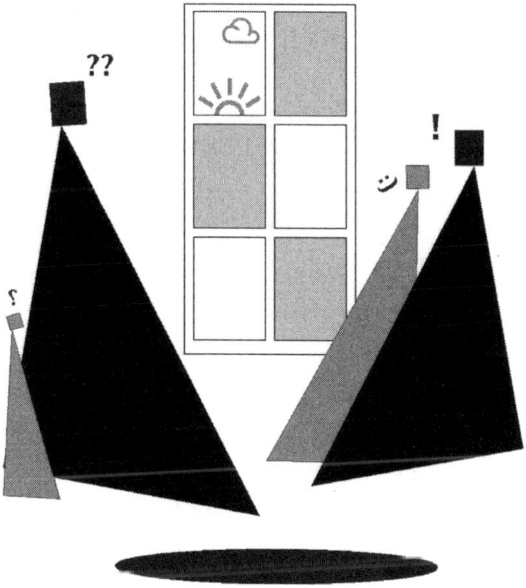

expectations.

Further research by Maccoby and Martin has suggested that a fourth parenting style could be added.[8]

Indifferent: Parents who are indifferent set few limits, hardly monitor the child's behaviour and are somewhat detached. Their children turn out to be demanding and less compliant, and tend to have poor peer relationships.

Barbara Coloroso, in *Kids are worth it!* introduces imagery which is different from that of Diana Birbaum. 'Authoritarian' becomes 'brickwall', 'indulgent' or 'permissive' turns into 'jellyfish' and 'authoritative' is called 'backbone'.[9]

This quote by Rudolf Steiner, an Austrian philosopher and spiritual scientist, should always be remembered: 'Children learn not from what we say or do, but from who we are'.[10] Steiner also talks about the four temperaments and how the temperamental make-up of the parents (even teachers) affects the children.[11]

Then we have the relatively new styles of parenting, which are characterized by what is popularly known as *helicopter parents* or

CASE STUDY

One day while waiting for our turn in the studio, we got chatting with the young employees at WorldSpace about how our parents brought us up. One of them said that his father was too strict. He hated every minute he spent in his restrictive home and could not wait to leave the house. Another youngster jumped in to say that his parents were very strict too, but he was, in fact, grateful for the way they had brought him up. He felt that he would have taken to wrong ways if they had not been firm with him. Everyone was puzzled by how the two perceived of a strict upbringing so differently. As we continued talking, we realized that the second set of parents, though firm, also expressed their love for their children in small but important, non-materialistic ways. The father of the first person, on the other hand, was unexpressive and did not feel the need or probably lacked the capacity to share and demonstrate his feelings towards his son. This made all the difference.

over-protective parents. Such parents hover over their children, not allowing them to take risks. They include *tiger moms,* who fiercely decide every move they think the kids should make. The author of *Battle Hymn of the Tiger Mother*, Amy Chua,[12] who is a law professor at Yale and a self-described 'tiger mother', forced her seven-year-old daughter, Lulu, to practise the piano for hours on end—'right through dinner into the night', with no breaks for water or even the bathroom, until at last Lulu learned to play the piece.

Chua, a petite 48-year-old mother of now teenaged daughters says, 'To be perfectly honest, I know that a lot of Asian parents are secretly shocked and horrified by many aspects of western parenting,' including 'how much time westerners allow their kids to waste—hours on Facebook and computer games; and in some ways, how poorly they prepare them for the future,' she told Meredith Vieira on a talk show with a toss of her long hair. 'It's a tough world out there.'

Parenting in this era

Very often, children are blamed by their parents for turning out the way they are when it is actually the parents who had used unfavourable child-rearing practices. There is a commonly heard, but not entirely fair adage: 'There are no problem children—only problem parents.' Having said that, it is unfair for parents to be criticized for blaming the children because, as far as they know, they are doing the right thing by their children. They do have the best intentions. They are doing things to the best of their knowledge and awareness. Unfortunately, children do not come with any instruction manuals on the best ways to raise them. Parents normally learn from their own parents, irrespective of whether their parents used good or unfavourable practices. Somehow it is hammered into their consciousness that what their parents said and did was the right thing. 'Parents can never be wrong' is the common belief. So they continue what their parents used to do. It is an understatement to say that the conditions in which they grew up were different from those in which their children are growing up. There are no more joint families, there are no more siblings and there is no support from grandparents. Children were not the centre of the parents' universe as they are today. Children used to grow up on their own among half a dozen siblings and cousins. They had to fend for themselves most of the time. There was no scope for throwing temper tantrums unless you were the last child, say, a son born after about six daughters!

Now many children are alone most of the time. Parents try to substitute their presence with expensive toys and babysitters. There are no role models. The child grows up watching television and playing violent games on the computer, and there is no one to monitor the content. Bringing up children is an entirely different experience in this day and age. Children today are growing up in a world of instant gratification and information overload. Distractions are too many. If parents expect their children to have the qualities that they had, or obey them at the slightest indication, then their expectations are not realistic. How will children obey parents who are not around most of the time? How will children know what to do when the rules are not consistent? It has never been tougher being a parent. But the important thing is to raise secure kids. Clear limits or dos and don'ts are necessary. Parents should make sure that rules are being followed and consequences must be inevitable if they are not followed. Not necessarily in the tiger mom style, but in a gentle, firm loving way that shows who is the boss.

Inconsistency

Take the example of a mother who goes to work. She picks up her child from the creche after work and goes back home tired. She still has to cook dinner. The child wants to see something on television that is not very suitable. If she changes the channel, he howls. Just to buy peace of mind, she agrees to something that she would never have agreed to had she had enough energy. Now she can at least finish cooking peacefully!

The mother chose the *easy way over the right way.* This leads to inconsistency of discipline. Inconsistency leads to a sense of insecurity in the child because there is the anxiety of not knowing when it is okay to do something and when it is not okay to do the same thing. (The child may unexpectedly get punished for something he was allowed to do only day before!)

There is another dimension to inconsistency. Imagine a situation in which the mother is trying to set ground rules. The father, or grandparents, who see very little of the child, would like to see the child happy, so they tell the mother to take it easy and try not to make the child cry. The result is that all the mother's efforts to try to discipline the child are wasted in one stroke. What is worse, the father often takes the child's side and even admonishes the mother in the child's presence. In this scenario, what respect will the child have for his mother? Will he ever listen to her again? You will even find him talking to his mother in the same tone as the father uses with her, as the father looks on at once amused and proud of his son.

What we are attempting to convey here is that parenting is not an instinctual knowledge. It is a science and also an art that needs to be learnt. A lot of research is being conducted in this area, and as mentioned above, researchers have come up with what seems to work and what does not. Parents have more access to information than ever before. They can obtain advice on how to raise children from the internet, magazines, newspapers, television, self-help books, workshops conducted by experts, etc. It is up to the parents to find out what works for them and what does not.

Goodness of fit

Every parent–child relationship is different and very personal as it is based on the interaction between two individuals, each of whose personality make-up is unique. That is why we see a difference between the way the same child relates to his father and to his mother, and how a mother relates to her two children (even twins). This is where the eternal debate between *nature versus nurture* comes into the picture. It is not just how parents discipline their child, but the inherent personality with which the child is born—his hereditary make-up—which determines the nature of the disciplining techniques that need to be adopted by the parents.

Some children are easy to deal with. They never trouble the parents in any way, they eat well and sleep well, on their own. Then there are other children born with a difficult temperament. They are cranky, whiny, easily angered and demanding.

The first category of children can be easily disciplined. The mother can control the child's every move with just a stern look. But with the second category of children, no amount of scolding, hitting, punishing or locking-up seems to work.

An example of a bad fit is the combination of a docile mother and a strong-willed child. In this case, the child may end up controlling the mother. The mother, too, wants to control the child and thus it becomes an eternal power struggle. The mother tries to compensate for her weak personality by trying to exert force on the child instead of using firmness and setting limits, which would actually take less effort and help the child respect his mother. When a mother is afraid that she is unable to 'control' the child as good mothers are supposed to, she becomes anxious, and the child, who can sense this anxiety, will take advantage, play around with this anxiety and manipulate the mother with all kinds of tactics.

There is, however, no need to despair. Problems arise due to lack of skills. These skills can be learnt. Methods of parenting, which affirm the dignity and humanity of both parents and children, are available for the asking.

When the problem goes beyond our control

The behaviour of a child is a radar of what is going on inside. There are signals that show us if the child is sad or happy, well-adjusted or if he is having a problem. Most children are either unable or afraid to talk about their state of mind. They try to cope with it in their own way. Their behaviour, verbal and non-verbal, is the only way in which they try to communicate their feelings. Unfortunately, their signals for help often go unnoticed, as parents and teachers are unaware of what a child's behaviour could mean. There may be a sudden drop in grades, which is usually the first sign; withdrawn behaviour, irritability, disobedience, frustration, and sleep and appetite disturbances when the child is going through a rough patch. Among the things that could be disturbing the child are the birth of a new baby, unmet needs, poor role models, bad company, unfavourable comparisons, learning problems, domestic violence and death or separation.

Parents and teachers label the child as a 'problem child' without attempting to explore the reasons behind his behaviour. Even

> *If there is anything that we wish to change in the child, we should first examine it and see whether it is not something that could better be changed in ourselves.*
>
> —C.G. JUNG, *Integration of the Personality*, 1939

a small, quiet talk may reveal what is bothering the child, but no such attempt is made. The child is shamed, humiliated, belittled and punished or 'disciplined', so to speak, making his behaviour go from bad to worse, until the parents suddenly realize that professional help is required.

When to seek professional help

- When parents feel they have tried everything and nothing seems to work
- When the problem interferes with the normal functioning of the child, such as his academic performance, appetite and sleep
- When the child seems to have unexplained fears and nightmares
- When the child suddenly complains of stomach aches, nausea, headaches, etc.
- When the child's problem starts having an impact on the other family members.

Positive approaches to disciplining

Parents should spend quality and fun time with their children, and demonstrate warmth and love. Once in a while, they should let go and let out their silly side.

- Discipline means 'loving authority'. Discipline never yields the expected results unless accompanied by love.
- The purpose of discipline is to channelize energy in a positive way.

- Set firm and consistent limits, and be clear about what the child can or cannot do. A child who grows up not knowing his limits will be an insecure child.
- Children learn by imitation and observation. The only way to discipline our children is to begin by disciplining ourselves. We need to walk the talk. We cannot yell and say, 'Don't yell!' We cannot expect our children to do something when they see that we are not doing it ourselves. We need to set standards and stick to them.
- Children expect consistent behaviour, routines and rhythms during the day, week and month as that will help them to know what to expect next and also what is expected of them. This gives them a sense of security.
- Recognize positive behaviour and appreciate the child's efforts. Praise the child generously, but honestly.
- Treat your child the way you want to be treated. Set good examples.
- Walk away and take some time off when you feel you are going to lose control. Do not say or do something that you may regret later.
- Talk to your child. Explain the consequences of both desirable and undesirable behaviour, and make sure you implement those consequences. Accept and acknowledge your children's opinions and feelings.
- Follow the right path, not the easy or convenient one.
- Paying attention only to unwanted behaviour actually increases it. Criticism or negative attention is also rewarding for children. They prefer getting scolded to being ignored. *Behaviour rewarded is behaviour repeated.*
- Do not give them choices. Choices can be confusing for young children. We need to demonstrate that we are the decision-makers. All the talk about parents being friends is all very well, but children need parents who will set limits for them, with whom they can feel free to communicate, from whom they can seek support and whom they can count on.

- Most importantly, we need to realize that our well-being has a direct impact on the well-being of our children. Children need parents who are calm, composed, balanced and well adjusted. None of us is perfect, but it is important for us to choose what we want to be and then keep trying. We may falter, we may fail, but then we know which path we have to get back on.

> The more fundamental issue is whether children are to be disciplined. The current debate has substituted the practice of 'positive discipline' of children in the place of corporal punishment. Although the elements of positive discipline emphasize interaction with children, respecting them and not punishing them, it is still within the bounds of a structure of authority of the teacher (parent) of the child. There is an undercurrent of acceptance that children need to be disciplined and told how to behave. This again positions the teacher (parent) and the child in an unequal relationship. It is important that the vocabulary used in this context changes to express equality in the relationship. Thus, a more apt concept is the use of 'positive engagement' of the teacher (parent) with the children.
>
> (From the Fourth Zakir Husain Memorial Lecture, 'Right to education and banning corporal punishment once and for all' by Professor Shantha Sinha, Chairperson, National Commission for Protection of Child Rights)

{ Chapter 4 }

Hyperparenting

Do not ask that your kids live up to your expectations. Let your kids be who they are, and your expectations will be in breathless pursuit.

—ROBERT BRAULT

'Look at your classmate—aren't both of you in the same class? If he can score 95%, why can't you? At this rate, all your classmates will be in engineering or medicine and you'll be working as a clerk in some bank. I have to push you now because I won't be able to do anything once you've already spoilt your life.' These days this must be a common dialogue heard in every household with an adolescent.

With more and more parents opting for one child or a maximum of two children, all the attention, hopes and ambitions of the parents are pinned on these poor children.

The following are some of the common parental attitudes towards children:

- The children are expected to fetch a reputation for the family. It is a status symbol if the child is an IIT or IIM graduate. The prevalent attitudes are reflected in phrases such as, '*Apne mata-pita ka naam roshan karo* (Bring good repute to your parents)' and, '*Hamara naam mitti mein mat milao* (Don't bring us discredit)'.
- The children are expected to make up for the failures and shortcomings of their parents. The parents seek redemption through their children for everything that has eluded them.
- The parents feel that how their children do in life will reflect on what kind of parents they are.
- Some parents expect that their children should take care of them

when they grow old. Parenting for them is a kind of investment. The more they push, the more secure their future will be!

Let us look at what happens stage by stage.

Infancy and toddlerhood

With schools coming up with programmes for toddlers, the pushing now starts in infancy. Mother and child can do activities together. Special CDs are designed for infants. If these programmes are designed keeping in mind the developmental readiness of the babies, there is no problem; it may even turn out to be beneficial to the child. But the trouble sets in when parents start pushing the child when he or she is not yet *developmentally ready* for it. For instance, children are admitted into pre-schools at the age of 2½.

Parents want their toddlers to get into the most elitist and posh schools of the city. They stand in queue from 4 a.m. to obtain applications for these schools. There is no problem with that either. However, in many cities, these schools conduct 'entrance exams' for children to get into lower kindergarten! And what do they test? The child's ability to write, if you please, and that, too, in cursive! If the child is already supposed to know how to write in cursive before he is granted admission, then what is it that they are going to teach?

Parents put their children into pre-schools and play homes, and put pressure on teachers to teach them cursive writing. If the schools do not do so, they will lose a customer to another school that does. This is where the competition begins, which continues throughout life.

The key aspect of the theory of Jean Piaget,[13] arguably the most scientific student of cognitive development, and who has been a major influence in curriculum planning for early childhood education, is the 'readiness of the child' for various activities. For example, a child cannot write till he is 5 years old, so forcing or pushing him to write earlier will only do more harm than good. The result may be that the child will tire too quickly of writing, and by the time he is 7–10 years old, he will develop an aversion to writing, or even develop writing problems at a later age. In clinical practice, one often finds that children who come in with some form of learning difficulty have been 'hurried children', that is, pushed before they are ready. They are pushed in a faulty way without being prepared with readiness skills that are usually imparted in some alternative methods of teaching such as the Waldorf and Montessori systems.

In Waldorf schools worldwide, reading and writing are not introduced until grade one. In kindergarten, teachers build upon the children's readiness skills.

That there is a natural sequence to be followed in understanding various concepts has been almost proven beyond doubt by Piaget. To try to get a child to appreciate the concept of density before he has understood the concept of conservation of volume is an effort doomed to failure. Similarly, before children can start counting, they must be familiar with the concepts of quantity and value. Children are like sponges. They absorb everything that is given to them; even the most abstract of concepts like the alphabet. But how long is a building without foundation going to last? Our children are turning into memorizing machines rather than human beings who can think originally and come up with creative solutions.

Primary and middle school

John Holt warned, 'We think badly, and even perceive badly, or not at all, when we are anxious or afraid... when we make children afraid, we stop learning dead in its tracks.'

This is what is induced in children from the beginning. Learning in most schools is reduced to mere marks and grades. Education is reduced to unit tests and quarterly examinations. No learning is applied to real life. 'Education' does not really teach how things work in real life. In today's context, education has been reduced to learning the particular answer given by the teacher to a particular question by rote.

Learning, which is actually a natural and enjoyable process for children from birth, is made to be associated with performance anxiety. 'If you don't get 90%, you are no good. Your value is weighed in terms of your marks.' Today's child does not know what the joy of learning is. He carries the drudgery of boring homework.

Added to this, children are forced to attend various classes after school. There are some who are kept busy every evening, with tennis, music, dance, badminton, abacus, or a myriad other classes, followed by homework. So much so that some of them have no time for play! Come holidays and they are made to attend activity-packed summer camps, some of which last all day, with the kids being dropped back only in the evening. When mothers get together, discussing whose child goes to how many classes makes interesting conversation.

Having said that, there are a handful of alternative schools in the country that attempt to understand how children learn best. The children passing out from these schools may not be top mark scorers, but they come out having confidence in their capabilities and knowing exactly what they want to do with their lives.

Parents need to know that to learn something, the child needs to be happy and enjoy it. Once the child is 8 or 9 years old, he can choose what he wants to learn. But do not be alarmed; children always seem to lose interest in a particular class after the initial excitement even if it is an activity of their own choice. If they have an aptitude, they will continue; if not, they have their ways of letting you know. Also, it is not very conducive for the healthy development of children to put them into structured classes at very young ages, especially under the age of 7.

According to physicians, if a child is pushed into a sport before he is physically and emotionally ready for it, his risk of injury increases. Let sports be fun. Putting too much focus on winning can make your child push too hard and risk injury.

High school

This is a different issue altogether and is of a much more serious nature, owing to the repercussions that the rat race at this stage has on young minds. Every year, a number of school and college kids commit suicide, either because they fail or fear they will fail their examinations. And often, the case is closed with the excuse that these were hypersensitive kids who could not handle the pressure. The parents' role in these cases is never questioned and lessons are never learnt from these experiences. Every year the number of children whose lives are nipped in the bud only seems to be increasing.

More and more youngsters are visiting psychiatrists and counsellors every year with high levels of stress and anxiety just a few months before examinations. The need of the hour is for schools to conduct workshops for students from Class 9 onwards, on topics such as:

- Stress management
- Goal-setting
- Time management
- Career planning
- Effective study skills.

This would enable and empower students to take charge of their lives, rather than crumble under pressure. Such classes would equip them with the skills required to face challenges and tackle pressure. There are positive steps being taken with the help of the media, to sensitize parents, to motivate students to seek help and to convince students that there is more to them than just a report card.

In most cases, parents take it upon themselves to decide their children's choice of career. The children's interest, choice or aptitude is never considered. Thousands of youngsters vie for a rank in the CET and other entrance examinations and think they have lost everything if they do not get it. Businessmen are cashing-in on this desperation to get into IITs and engineering colleges and charging high fees and offering paid seats for medicine and engineering. Parents pay lakhs of rupees for something for which the child may not even have the aptitude! Of course, there are also the numerous coaching classes which are minting money.

This is where Howard Gardner and his theory of multiple intelligences come in.[14] 'It is not important to know how much is the intelligence of a child, but it is important how the child is intelligent', says Ratnesh Mathur, founder of Genie Kids, an activity centre in Bengaluru based on the multiple intelligence theory of Howard Gardner. Howard Gardner is a professor at Harvard University and the author of many books, including *Frames of Mind*. His theory of multiple intelligences has challenged long-held assumptions about intelligence, especially about a single measure of intelligence.

The original seven intelligences

It is in *Frames of Mind* that Howard Gardner first identified and introduced us to seven different kinds of intelligence. These are—linguistic, logical–mathematical, musical, spatial, bodily–kinesthetic, interpersonal and intrapersonal. Gardner then identified an eighth intelligence, the naturalist intelligence. For example, Zakir Hussain is musically intelligent, Tendulkar's intelligence is of a bodily–kinesthetic kind (yes, he is intelligent even if he is a school drop-out, and thank God his parents had the good sense to realize that), and Charles Darwin's was naturalistic intelligence.

Thanks to Gardner, teachers can have an understanding of every child's learning style and can make learning a more interesting process in the classroom. Children can also choose careers based on their specific intelligence. Parents are requested to find out the way in which the child is intelligent and where his interest lies before blindly pushing him to prepare for IIT. Is A.R. Rahman not making money? Is Ritu Beri not making money? Are people in advertising and photography not making money? They are not only making money, but are also enjoying their work. Now how many people can

CASE STUDIES

Mrs M, the mother of two boys, one three years old and the other seven years old, sends them to dance classes and is grooming them for a dance reality show. They perform suggestive adult moves with the ease with which children act out nursery rhymes.

The mother of a child who was on the autism spectrum was, like many others, anxious to make the best use of the time available and would take him from school to therapy after therapy. The child had almost no time to relax. One day, he reached breaking point and cried for a full two days. His doctor instructed his mother to stop all therapies. He asked her to just spend time with him at home for a few days and maybe take him to the park to relax and play. After that wake-up call, she realized that he was a child first and no child deserves to be subjected to so much pressure. She decided to send him for only the most essential therapies.

This district is notorious for starting the kids early, for example, as early as the 6th grade for IIT coaching. The children go to a day boarding school, where they stay back after school hours up to 9 p.m. to be coached for the IIT entrance examination. It is 9:30 p.m. by the time they reach home. They have just enough time to eat a quick dinner and go to sleep. Many of these children who make it to IIT take to drugs and resort to other less desirable ways to deal with pressure.

The year 2012 saw the launch of a fashion week for children's designer fashion. The children were walking the ramp in revealing clothes not meant for children.

These are true stories. Do children have a childhood any more? Will these children ever know what they want to do with their own life rather than being sources of wish-fulfilment for their parents?

boast of that? If people are forced into careers for which they have no aptitude, they may burn out before they reach their optimum potential. But if they like what they do, or do what they like, no one can stop them from achieving greater heights. (Having said that, are we assuming that earning lots of money guarantees happiness?)

One of the major aims of the Waldorf education system is to help the child find out who he is and his true purpose in life. 'Our highest endeavour must be to develop free human beings who are able by themselves to impart purpose and direction to their lives', Rudolf

Here are some tips to help your children have a strong belief in themselves and excel in everything they do:

- Praise them for little achievements and mighty efforts, even if they do not succeed.
- Avoid shaming them and making them feel guilty for what they have not achieved. It will not help them do better the next time.
- Focus on how much they have improved over their last performance. Do not dwell on how much less they have got than the others. Let their own past performance be the sole point of comparison.
- Encourage them in areas in which they are good. This confidence will spread to all areas of their lives and enhance their performance.
- Pay full attention when they are talking to you.
- Keep communication channels open and encourage them to express their feelings. Listen with empathy. By not doing so, you will not be able to find out about their feelings, conflicts and what is bothering them until it is too late.
- Give them all the support and understanding that they need to be able to deal with failure.

Steiner, the founder of Waldorf education, said.

A psychology professor said recently: 'Parents should not bombard children with multiple inputs to transform them into super child role models. It is not about showcasing their parenting skills, but about the child's healthy growth.'

Sending children for too many classes stifles their creativity. They need time and space to explore the world in their own way, let their imagination grow and find out what holds their interest the most.

{ Section III }

RELATIONSHIP ISSUES

{ Chapter 5 }

Parent–Child Relationships

Children begin by loving their parents; as they grow older they judge them; sometimes they forgive them.

—OSCAR WILDE

When you think of the phrase parent–child relationship, what do you visualize? Do you see a mother and child tucked in a warm bed with book in hand, or do you see the imposing figure of a parent towering over a little child, one hand on the hip and the other pointing accusingly at the child? Or do you see a little child riding on his dear dad's back, saying, 'Giddy up horsy!'? What you will visualize depends on the kind of childhood you had, or the kind of childhood you would have liked to have.

The kind of parents we are to our children depends on the kind of parents we had. It is paradoxical that most of us who have suffered at the hands of our parents do not think, 'I have suffered, I will not let my child suffer…,' but instead, tend to pass on that suffering because that is the only way we know.

This is exactly what happens in cases of child abuse—physical, emotional or sexual. Most abusers have most likely themselves been abused as children. Very few people, like Dave Pelzer, a child abuse victim and the best-selling author of *A Child Called "It"* and *A Man Named Dave*, decide that they will be the one to stop the trend of abuse in the family lineage.[15]

When does the parent–child relationship begin? With a child's birth, of course, you may say. Actually, the relationship starts with the decision to have a baby. The following questions have a bearing on the relationship:

- Was the decision to have the baby a planned and conscious one? Or was it an unexpected or unwanted accident?
- Did one of the parents-to-be have unfavourable experiences as a child; for example, being the first born in a large family in which he/she had to take care of his/her younger siblings? Or was he/she an only child with a lonely childhood and desperately wants to have a baby of his/her own?
- Was the mother alone and unsupported with this new life growing in her?
- Was there an unsuccessful attempt to terminate the baby?
- Did the mother have the loving care of the father of the baby-to-be?
- Even if the conception was an accident, have the once-reluctant parents reconciled to this development and decided to approach it with a new, positive attitude?
- Did they fear whether or not they could be good parents?

The following questions are relevant once the decision is taken to continue with the pregnancy:

- During pregnancy, was the mother-to-be pampered and taken good care of? Or was she in a joint family, in which she was not only forced to do all the work, but did not even receive any special care?
- Did the mother resent having to lose her figure or her job?
- Did the father worry about the financial burdens of raising the child?
- How was the physical and mental health of the mother?

The seeds of the parents' attitudes towards the baby, and consequentially, of the baby's emotional development, are sown at this stage. The attitudes of not only the mother, but also of the father and the significant others in the family affect the just-formed foetus.

When parental attitudes, formed before the baby's birth, are favourable, they tend to persist after the baby's birth. This contributes to a good parent–child relationship. The mother's attitude can have an effect on her unborn baby, not just through the umbilical cord, but as a result of endocrinal changes which can and do occur if the mother-to-be is exposed to severe and prolonged stress during pregnancy. This kind of stress normally accompanies persistently unfavourable attitudes on the part of the mother towards the child when the pregnancy is sudden, unplanned or unwanted.

After birth, the mother's attitudes, most of which were formed before the baby's birth, have an influence because they are reflected in the way the child is treated. For example, a mother who wanted a boy will have a less favourable attitude towards a daughter. She may try to compensate for the feelings of guilt caused by this disappointment by being overprotective and overindulgent towards the child. If a later child should be the hoped-for son, then she may display favouritism towards the son.

Concepts of security and attachment[16]

John Bowlby formulated the basic tenets of the theory of Attachment. He said that to grow up mentally healthy 'the infant and young child should experience a warm, intimate and continuous relationship with his mother (or permanent mother-substitute) in which both find satisfaction and enjoyment'. He explained a child's ties to the mother and its disruption through separation, deprivation and bereavement. Mary Ainsworth's ideas not only helped in expanding the theory but also gave it new directions. Ainsworth introduced the concept of attachment as a secure base from which an infant can explore the world. She also formulated the concept of maternal sensitivity to infant signals and its role in the development of infant–mother attachment patterns.

Ainsworth said that familial security in the early stages is of a dependent type and forms a basis from which the individual can work out gradually, forming new skills and interests in other fields.

Where familial security is lacking, the individual is handicapped by the lack of what might be called a secure base. She found that securely attached infants cried little and seemed content to explore in the presence of mother; insecurely attached infants cried frequently, even when held by their mothers, and explored little; and not-yet attached infants manifested no differential behaviour to the mother. It is observed that when mothers mix their own playful behaviour with that of their babies, infants respond with joyful bouncing, smiling and vocalizing.

Knowing where we come from

All parents want the best for their children and are concerned with their well-being and happiness. At the same time, many parents find themselves limited to varying degrees in their ability to provide the love, warmth, direction and control necessary for their child's optimal emotional development.

Besides the pressure of balancing work and family responsibilities, the most significant problems we all face in raising children can be traced to our families of origin. In order to be effective parents and develop secure attachments with our children, we need to make sense of what happened in our own childhood. By recognizing where our beliefs and feelings about children come from, we can gain more control over the defensive behaviour that we feel compelled to act out with our children.

Parents try various methods and techniques to bring about changes and improvements in their children. If these methods do not first bring about a change in the parents themselves in terms of lifestyle or attitude, they are unlikely to bring about any change in the children. Our attitudes and beliefs are reflected in the way our children deal with various situations in life. The ambivalent attitudes we have towards ourselves are inevitably extended to our feelings about our children.

What is the most important thing a person can do to be the best possible parent?

We can best help our children by trying to fulfil our own lives. When we are involved in an honest pursuit of our own development, we serve as positive role models for our children. Learning to have compassion for ourselves enables us to extend that compassion to our children. According to Robin Sharma, the author of *Family Wisdom*, the best way to become a better parent is by first becoming a better person.[17]

Ways to nurture parent–child relationships

Just as with any relationship, building a positive relationship between parent and child requires work and effort. Only then can the relationship be strong and successful. Parenting is a tough job, and maintaining a close relationship and open communication channels helps to ensure that the parents and their child stay connected through all ages of their upbringing. Some simple tips for enhancing the bond between parent and child are discussed below.

Say 'I love you'

Tell your child every day that you love him, no matter what his age. Even on difficult days or after a disagreement with the child, when you do not exactly 'like your child' (i.e. 'do not like what he did') at that moment, it is important, in fact, more important than ever, to express your love. A simple 'I love you' goes a long way towards developing and strengthening a relationship. It shows that you disapprove of what he did but not him as such.

Warmth towards the child can be expressed not only through the spoken word, but also through actions and gestures, such as a pat on the back or ruffling of the hair. We can express our love for them through our mere presence when they need us.

Some parents do not show any kind of feelings towards their children (ambivalence). They may feel that it is all right not to show positive feelings as long as they do not show negative feelings towards the child. Expression of feelings is very difficult for them and comes only with great effort, and they are uncomfortable doing it.

As the famous saying goes, 'Love me, hate me, but don't ignore me.' All that children need is attention—positive or negative. When parents pay attention only to undesirable behaviour and do not remember to acknowledge positive behaviour, they unwittingly become responsible for maintaining the child's negative behaviour. Remember, behaviour rewarded, whether with positive or negative attention, is behaviour repeated. It is believed that children are happy to get even negative attention. Not paying any attention at all is worse than giving negative attention.

Teach your faith

Teach your child about your faith, values and beliefs. Tell him what you believe and why. Allow your child the time to ask questions and answer them honestly. Reinforce those teachings often. Grab the magical moments that come along once in a while when you find your child receptive to whatever you say, and impart your life's lessons in those moments.

Touch

According to one study, touch is the most important sensory stimulation that a parent can give a child. Hugs, cuddles, kisses (even teenagers enjoy being cuddled!), pats on the back, ruffling their hair, simply holding their hand and other affectionate gestures speak louder than words when it comes to showing how you feel about your child. (This works very well for us adults, too.)

Develop and maintain a special bedtime ritual

For younger children, reading a favourite bedtime book or telling stories is a ritual that the child will most likely remember throughout his life. Older children should not be neglected either. Once children start reading, have them read a page, chapter or short book to you. Even most teenagers still enjoy the ritual of being told goodnight in a special way by a parent.

Let your children help you

Parents sometimes inadvertently miss out on opportunities to forge closer relationships by not allowing their child to help them with various tasks and chores. Unloading groceries after going to the store is a good example of something that children of most ages can and should assist with. Choosing which shoes look better with your dress lets a child know you value his opinion. Of course, if you ask, be prepared to accept and live with the choice made!

Play with your children

You should make sure you play with your children. Play with dolls or a ball, indulge in make-believe, play checkers, involve the child in sing-songs, or do whatever is fun and interesting. It does not matter what you play, just enjoy each other! Let the kid see your silly side. Older kids enjoy cards, chess and computer games, while younger ones will have fun playing with anything, as long as it involves you!

Eat meals as a family

You have heard this before, and it really is important. Eating together sets the stage for conversation and sharing. Turn the television off, and do not rush through a meal. Talk and enjoy each other's company. Meal-times can constitute quality time, a time that will be remembered for long after by children and parents alike.

Seek out one-on-one opportunities

Some parents have special nights or 'standing dates' with their children to create one-on-one opportunities. Whether it is a walk around the neighbourhood, a special trip to a playground or a night at the movies with just the two of you, it is important to celebrate each child individually. Although creating one-on-one opportunities is more of a challenge if there are many children in a family, it is actually achievable. Think creatively and the opportunities created will be ones that you will remember in the future.

Respect their choices

You do not have to like your child's mismatched shirt and shorts or love how he has placed pictures in his room. However, it is important to respect those choices. Children look for independence at a young age, and parents can help to foster their decision-making skills by being supportive and even looking the other way on occasion. After all, it really does not matter if a child goes to picnic with a striped green shirt and pink shorts. Having said that, they do not deserve the burden of having too many choices either.

Make them a priority in your life

Your children need to know that you believe they are a priority in your life. They can observe excessive stress and notice when you are not paying them attention.

Report your child's achievements, efforts and good qualities

When you talk proudly of your child's efforts, achievements and qualities to your spouse or any other person, you can see your child glow with pride and joy. Such acknowledgement will give his morale a big boost and give him the impetus to try harder next time. This, in turn, will go a long way in increasing his self-confidence.

Empathize and demonstrate concern

When your child comes back sulking from school, do not smother him with a hundred questions. Try to show that you understand his feelings and he will himself tell you what is bothering him, if he wants to. If he does not, leave him alone. The knowledge that you are there to listen to him, that you empathize, and that you care for and respect his feelings will help him to trust you. For example, when he walks in sulking, say, 'You look upset' and leave it at that. When he tells you something like, 'I feel like bashing up that chemistry teacher,' do not jump in with, 'That's no way to talk about your teachers!' Instead, try saying, 'My, my, he's really upset you today,' or 'You are that angry with him?' Then the child will understand that you really understand and want to help. If you dismiss the child's feelings, the conversation will end right there and you will lose an opportunity to bond with him.

Listen actively

When your child comes enthusiastically to show you something he has created, do not dismiss him with a cursory glance and a perfunctory 'very nice'. The child will get the message that you are just saying it without actually meaning it. If you are reading your paper, put it down, look at his drawing for a minute and comment on a detail that really deserves to be appreciated; for example, 'Nice clouds', or 'How did you stick this?' or 'What colour pencils did you use?' The child will know that you are genuinely paying attention and will believe you. One girl was heard joking about her dad: 'When my dad is reading the newspaper and I go tell him, "Dad, I am jumping off the balcony," he's likely to say, "Oh unh-unh!"'[18]

Parental angst

More than fathers, mothers are often unable to experience joy in a parent–child relationship due to the anxiety involved in raising a child. Why do you think the teacher who is able to handle a class of 40 brats is able to maintain her cool, but gets impatient with her own child? Anxiety. She is not anxious about the children she teaches—not that she cares any less, but she is more objective when she is just a teacher.

Children are more receptive to people other than their mother when it comes to academics or learning some skill, because they sense their mother's anxiety. It makes them nervous.

Why are grandparents so much more relaxed with their grandchildren than they ever were with their own children? Because they are not anxious—anxious about whether they will fulfil their expectations. Parents worry about things such as how their children will turn out as adults, whether they are as good as their parents were at child-raising, and what will happen if they lose control over their child. Grandparents do not worry about these things and want to enjoy their grandchildren in a way that they could not enjoy their own children.

It will be great, if, once in a while, we remember the joy that we once felt when we held 'the bundle of joy' in our hands. It is the same bundle standing in front of us today as a defiant teenager. Is it possible for parents to enjoy their children just the way they are? Is it possible for us not to judge ourselves or our children? Is it possible for us to be conscious in the choices we make for our children, for ourselves? Choices that ring true in our heart, at least once in a while?

{ Chapter 6 }

The Generation Gap

First we are children to our parents, then parents to our children, then parents to our parents, then children to our children.

—MILTON GREENBLATT

Chennai, 1997

Mother to daughter: 'What is it that you're wearing? I can't let you go out in that figure hugging T-shirt. Go change!'

Chennai, 2011

Daughter to Mother: 'Ma! You're wearing my tee again! I told you not to go near my closet, didn't I?'

This is a typical urban scenario these days—figure-conscious mammas, armed with tools that help them to defy age and credit cards. Twenty years back, most Indian women wore only saris, but today things are different. The rate at which the world has been changing over the years is increasing. Say 70 years back, the generation gap meant a gap of 15 or 20 years; the gap is now a period of just five years! This gap exists, but it seems to be decreasing.

What is the generation gap?

'A difference in attitudes between people of different generations, leading to lack of understanding.'[19] Barker defines the term as: 'The differences in values, lifestyles and economic opportunities that exist between people of different age cohorts living in the same society.'[20] It is something that has bothered parents and teenagers for generations... us, our parents and their parents. It seems like a mystery that has been puzzling all of us.

Two aspects are to be considered when we talk about the generation gap. Firstly, it is the gap between parents and children and secondly, the differences between how parents and children were earlier and how they are now. These two aspects often overlap. So while we say that the world is changing rapidly, the gap between parents and children is also decreasing.

The generation gap has existed since time immemorial. However, the term first came into prominence in western countries during the 1960s and described the *cultural differences* between the baby boomers and their parents. Although history had always witnessed some degree of generational differences, during the 1960s the differences between the two generations were significantly magnified in comparison to those in previous times. There were major differences in such matters as tastes in music and fashion, drug use and politics. This situation may have been accelerated by the unprecedented size of the young baby boomer generation, which gave these people a greater sense of power and influence than had been seen previously, and the younger generation was willing to rebel against societal norms to a degree not seen before.

The generation gap is far more than the wildness of youth. It is basically a war between cultures, or the friction between people who do not understand each other.

Comparing the generations

In the 1920s, youngsters learned of cars and machines, whereas their parents had travelled by horseback or by foot, or had not travelled at all. Trips across the world became possible almost on a whim, though this did not become popular until another generation had passed and

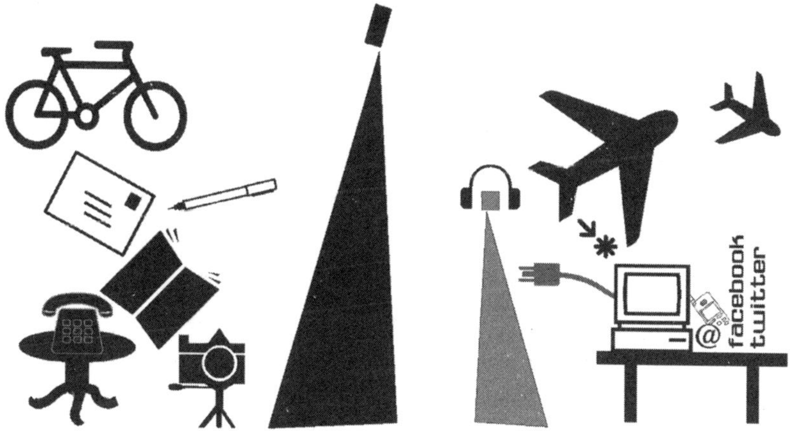

the idea could seem 'normal'; normal to a new generation that grew up with cars.

In the 1950s, television made its appearance, but it was not until a generation later that everyone was hooked. In the late 1970s and early 1980s, the electronic age was just beginning, as we turned to computers. Today's children are so casual about computers. While their parents looked upon computers as serious business, today's children live in the virtual world of gaming, Facebook and Twitter to the exclusion of everyone and everything else!

Changing or diminishing values

'The generation gap exists today and we can see it in the form of changing values', says Apeksha, 45, a mother of two teenagers. With the family structure changing rapidly, the role of the elder members of extended families is diminishing. Grandparents were previously the ones who maintained family values and traditions and who passed them down to the next generation. Today, children tease their grandparents for being out of time if they do not learn how to use mobile phones or send emails. These changing priorities have made all the wisdom of the older generation passé and those who are 'tech-savvy' are valued. So grandparents, who are not so old any more (sixties are the new forties, remember?), have their own Facebook pages and keep in touch with their relatives abroad, with whom they would have lost touch otherwise!

The generation gap is more of an urban phenomenon. Rural India is still too busy struggling with day-to-day life to be affected by such matters, and human relationships still mean a lot. The erosion of old values is especially evident in urban settings, in which more and more children are left all to themselves at home after school. They spend most of their time surfing the net, to which they have free access, and watching American TV sitcoms and music channels. Urban children are being exposed to content which may not be appropriate for their age or culture. They are learning too much too soon and not necessarily the right thing in the right way. Children as young as ten are talking about homosexuality with utter casualness. There is no monitoring of what they are doing and absorbing, and technology is babysitting the children of the present generation.

Female foeticide still takes place and gender bias still exists, but the emancipation of women has definitely begun. Girls are getting higher education and are excelling in their courses. They are competing with boys for the top jobs and are aggressively competitive. This has been great for women, but what effect is it having on the families, on the children and on the well-being of women themselves?

The upside is that men have started sharing in the family responsibilities and child-rearing. Fathers know more about their children today than they did 25 years ago. Women have more freedom to go out and earn, and also realize their potential.

The downside is that mothers still have the major portion of the responsibility of child-care. If the child falls sick, it is still the mother who takes the day off. She still has to manage the house and host dinners and parties. She also has to take care of the bank work, school meetings and grocery shopping. The woman of today has much more on her plate than she ever had before. She is constantly juggling and tightrope-walking in her effort to balance her various roles. There is too much pressure on her and she is perpetually stressed.

With both parents joining the workforce, and with today's women having much more to do than only taking care of the home and children, more and more urban children are growing up in the care of maids, in day-care centres or in front of the television and computers, which has eroded their link with the older generation and its traditions and values. We ought to focus on measures which would ensure that the grandparents or parents remain responsible for the various nurturing and educational functions required to maintain and support their children in every way.

The results of a Nickelodeon survey (2007), however, reveal something different. In this survey, 80% of young people named their parents and 19% named their grandparents as the people they admired the most.[21] Recent research has found that feelings of connectedness with the family, other adults, the community and social institutions greatly contribute to the health of the youth.

According to another study, there were fewer instances of drug use, delinquency and sexual precociousness among children belonging to families that followed the tradition of having their dinner together.

The generation gap and adolescence

It is more or less smooth sailing for parents until their children enter the tempestuous phase of adolescence. This is the time when children are trying to form a new identity, coming out of the dependence of childhood and moving into the independence and the accompanying insecurity of adulthood. This is when parents need to strike a balance between control and freedom, which is no easier than doing a tightrope walk across the Niagara. Building trust is of vital importance in this phase. 'There is a generation gap between me and my teenage son, but I feel better when I can recollect something similar in my own teens. But one can understand since times are different and influences are different', says Geetha, 48, empathizing with her son.

Some parents, who sway towards the freedom side of the balance, need to realize that if they were to throw in the towel and let their teenagers run wild without any supervision, it would be a truly frightening experience for their children. Teenagers may not know it or admit it, but they need their parents to guide them on what is right and what is wrong. In dealing with an adolescent, age does matter and no matter how things change, parents should go with their instincts when it comes to deciding that some things are just not done.

'The main difference I see between me and my son is that I used to fear my father and dared not argue even if what he said was wrong. I would just do what he expected. But my son never hesitates to tell me that he knows what he is doing and that I should let him be. If he is talking so boldly, I am responsible for it because I did not want my son to grow up in fear. At the same time, I know my son is capable of making the right choices and taking care of himself because I do tell him what is right and wrong and leave it at that. I am careful not to nag him', says Amit, who is a long-distance parent.

Drugs, sexuality and the internet were not a concern for our parents when we were growing up. Just as our society has followed in the footsteps of the West with the dissolution of the joint family, career-oriented mothers and increasing divorce rates, our children are now experimenting with sex and drugs. However, teenagers in the West have gone full circle and are now talking about abstinence (heard of the abstinence ring?) in a big way, while our teenagers are just trying out the things that their western counterparts are now trying to abandon.

Adolescence is the time when teenagers try to become individuals in their own right and try to move out from under the protective wing of their parents. They will try out many things in order to be 'in' with the crowd, whether it is smoking, drinking, wearing skimpy clothes or even losing their virginity.

In 2005, there was a much-publicised controversy about a south Indian actor's remarks in an interview for AIDS awareness, about the need for protected sex.[22] She said it was fine for girls to have pre-marital sex, but not without taking precautions to prevent pregnancy and sexually transmitted infections. Later, she added that no educated man should expect his wife or girlfriend to be a virgin. Political parties condemned her statement and she was taken to court, but the Supreme Court dismissed all charges against her. This controversy made people somewhat aware of the reality of premarital sex in the light of the AIDS scenario. It served as a wake-up

Communication with your adolescent child is essential. The way to deal with him is not by making yourself out to be the enemy and coming down on him heavily for every transgression (and there will be many).

- Try to lay down the ground rules right in the beginning.
- Empathize with your children without judging their behaviour.
- Give them options that are, in the first place, acceptable to you, such as, 'Do you want to finish your studies before playing, or after?' When the child makes a choice that you have given, then do not say, 'I think it is better you finish studying first.'
- It is difficult for anyone to interpret the teenage mind, but try to convey the fact that you are on their side.
- Parents tend to forget that they, too, were teenagers once, and their self-righteousness does not win them any points with their children.
- Sit with them once in a while and share their joy in the books, films and music that they enjoy.
- Again, loving-authority is the key. Children are more accepting of our rules when we come across with love rather than control.
- Make it a point to have dinners together.

call to parents who assume their children will never get into trouble, to address safety issues nonetheless. Parents need to wake up to the fact that the average age at which children lose their virginity is decreasing even in India. It is important to equip them with life skills that are required for them to deal with such situations and help them make right choices. Most parents tend to forget that babies do grow up some day and when the time comes, they must let them go to find their own way in the world. You cannot protect your children forever and they will not thank you if you try to.

The most unrealistic mistake that parents make is to compare their teenagers to themselves when they were that age. It is unrealistic because the circumstances have changed. The culture has changed. The social mores have changed and our own lifestyles and values have changed since the time of our parents. Given this scenario, how can we expect our children to be like us?

The shrinking generation gap and new-age parenting

Research has shown that the maximum gap between parents and children existed in the late 1960s and early 1970s, globally. The gap has been gradually decreasing since then and is at its lowest now. Parents and children today dress alike, listen to the same music and are friends. Is this a good thing?

The upside

Sometimes, when Arun and his 16-year-old daughter, Ruchi, listen to rock music together and talk about pop culture—interests they both enjoy—Arun recalls his relationship with his parents when he was a teenager, a relationship which was more distant. In the past, the gulf was apparent not only in musical tastes. From clothing and hairstyles to activities and expectations, earlier generations of parents and children often appeared to revolve in separate orbits.

Today, the generation gap has not disappeared, but is shrinking in many families. The old authoritarian approach to discipline—a starchy 'because I said so, that's why'—is giving way to a new egalitarianism and a 'come, let us reason together' attitude. The result can be a rewarding closeness among family members. Conversations which would not have taken place a generation ago, or which would have been awkward, on subjects such as sex and drugs are comfortable and common today. Parent–child activities, from shopping to sports, involve an easy camaraderie that can continue into adulthood.

The downside

Family experts, however, caution that the new equality can also have a downside—diminishing respect for parents. In metros, it is increasingly seen that 40-something mothers dress up like their 20-something daughters. A fitness trainer from Delhi is quoted as saying that the eagerness to mimic the daughter has mostly to do with the mother's latent insecurities. There are women who insist on getting procedures such as breast firming, wrinkle removals, etc. to look like an 18-year-old. What they do not understand is that it is unnatural to look 18 when one is 40.

At another level, many parents have started making decisions on the basis of what their child wants. The power has shifted to children. Increasing guilt on the part of busy parents makes them less eager to spend time disciplining their children. Parents who are short of time also encourage their children to be independent, making them more responsible for themselves, which is a good thing, but they often compensate for lack of time with material gifts. Some parents worry that if they say 'no' to their child or impose limits, it will hurt the child's self-esteem.

Parents who do not set rules risk becoming so powerless in their own homes that they feel out of control. Parents have to be careful not to be totally their child's buddy, because they still have to be the parents who set the rules. There are also parents who, in their eagerness to keep the peace and avoid arguments, miss an opportunity to teach their children how to resolve conflicts, rather than simply avoiding them.

Problem of plenty

Today's growing middle and upper middle class is enjoying a new wave of consumerism. Companies are vying with each other with attractive offers. Banks are offering loans and credit cards. In spite of being aware of what happened not so long ago in the USA, people are falling into the credit trap. The invasion of the cities by the mall culture is turning us into big spenders. The invasion of television, with its serials and commercials, is seducing us into leading an unreal life, tempting us to spend on what we do not need. As a result, children have a problem of plenty. They have more than they need, even before they ask, and are yet always unsatiated, wanting more.

Excessive entertainment with television, laptops, phones and video-games has given rise to the new maladies of the 21st century—boredom and instant gratification. Aggressive marketing is prompting companies to produce snacks with more flavours, phones with more features, fast food joints with bigger servings and cosmetics with more chemicals.

This is a generation of excesses. When everyone is used to having an excess of everything assaulting their senses every second of their waking life, why would anyone want to settle for less? Normal is now boring. We are increasingly finding it difficult to live in the present moment and this is giving rise to learning problems among children and relationship problems among adults.

It is easy to unconsciously go with the flow and say, 'The whole world is like that! What can we do?', whereas the challenge is to stop, think, question whether we are making the right choices, and determine if this is essential and if this is good.

We need to strike a balance, with parents once again being viewed as parents, and not as peers to their children. Children are being viewed as very loved and valued family members, and their feelings are respected, but the power or authority should lie with the parents.

The best thing for the parents to do after reading all the self-help books and seeking all the help from the experts is to try and figure out what works best for them, their child and their family. Every person is different and there is no thumb rule in parenting. It is best to trust our own heart and our intuition. As long as we are not going against our conscience, we will do well for ourselves and our children.

{ Chapter 7 }

Sibling Rivalry

Sibling relationships outlast marriages, survive the death of parents, resurface after quarrels that would sink any friendship. They flourish in a thousand incarnations of closeness and distance, warmth, loyalty and distrust.

—ERICA E. GOODE

You may recall the biblical story of the two brothers, Cain and Abel, the children of Adam and Eve. Abel is a conscientious worker and Cain is laidback. When it is time for them to make offerings of their produce to God, Abel presents the best of his crop, while Cain, who is a shepherd, presents inferior offerings. When God accepts Abel's and rejects Cain's offerings, Cain, overpowered by anger and jealousy, slays his brother. The gospels preach that people should have brotherly love for each other, by which they mean that they should live harmoniously with each other. But is this harmony natural in a brotherly relationship?

What is sibling rivalry?

By 'sibling rivalry' we mean the antagonism or hostility between brothers and/or sisters, which ranges from the everyday fights between children in the family, e.g. one sibling pulling the other's hair or unwilling to share a prized toy—situations which test the patience of parents all over the world, to much more serious cases, such as permanent enmity between adult siblings due to matters such as property dealings.

Sibling rivalry is a normal and inevitable part of growing up. It normally starts with the birth of the second child, when the older one starts feeling neglected and possessive. The younger ones are at the receiving end most of the time because of the difference in size and capacity, but as they grow, they learn how to evade the older siblings' attacks and develop tactics to bother them. Often, adults end up taking the side of the young ones although the elder one may have been the victim.

I had my second daughter ten years after the first one. The older one took full advantage of the little one's smallness and had a lot of fun teasing her, and the little one used to bawl (perhaps a little more than was needed, knowing mom's tendency and need to protect her from the older one!).

When I desperately turned to my mentor for help, she calmly told me to leave them alone to sort out their past *karma* with each other! This helped me to be more objective and not take sides, though unwittingly it made matters worse. Today, the little one is a tough cookie who is capable of taking care of herself. My elder one prides herself in having trained her well (*see* Case Study, p. 80).

Manifestations

One of the forms of sibling rivalry is competitiveness. In fact, this can be seen even in animals and birds, with the stronger one overpowering the weaker ones and, in many instances, killing them, so that it can have the catch all for itself. Among humans, the competitiveness is for resources that are limited and precious—parents, and their love, attention and approval. Before the birth of the second child, the first child has been the centre of all attention and affection, and has been fussed over exclusively. Once the second child is born, this attention is divided between the two. The first one may get even less than half the attention as the newborn is so delicate and vulnerable. This is where the competition begins.

Sibling rivalry can be characterized by negative feelings, overt hostility, malicious behaviour, violence, undermining, reluctance to share and lack of positive regard for each other. Sometimes children

The common signs of a child having trouble with his new sibling are:

- There may be sudden complaints from the school teacher that this previously perfectly behaved child is acting up, disrupting class and troubling other children.
- The older one thinks that the parents and everybody likes his new sibling more. Due to insecurity and anxiety, the older one often starts regressing in his behaviour. Children who had gained bladder control start bedwetting again. Children who never sucked their thumbs start doing so. Children whose language was perfectly developed for their age suddenly start baby talking (often in imitation of the younger sibling).
- The child starts defying his parents, opposing everything that he is told. When this goes too far, it is called *oppositional defiance disorder*. The child sometimes starts using bad language, throws tantrums and even becomes disruptive, breaking and flinging things.
- There could be disturbances in sleep and appetite. The child may want the mother to feed him when she is feeding the baby or he may want to sleep next to the mother. His sleep may be disturbed and he may get up crying.
- The child may cry about going to school and may start clinging to the mother.

come up with scheming ways to make their siblings look bad, although they are the perpetrators.

Preparing the first child for a new baby

The process of adjusting to a new sibling need not be painful for either the child or the parents if the child is adequately prepared to receive the newcomer.

- The child must be prepared as early during pregnancy as possible for the new baby that will soon be a part of the family.
- The child will have to be informed that his mother will have to give the baby time, but that he will surely have his own exclusive time with his mother too, when they will share fun that the baby cannot be a part of.
- The child will have to be involved by being told that any help he can give in taking care of the baby will be important. He will have new responsibilities and these will change as he grows. However, at the same time, the parents must be careful not to put too many responsibilities on the child and must not have too many expectations. He may not be capable of fulfilling them, and since he would want to gain his parents' approval, he will feel defeated if he is not able to come up to their expectations.

Helping the mother may not be the only expectation from the child. He may also be expected to be understanding and not complain that he is not getting enough time. It must be remembered that even if the child is the baby's older brother or sister, he/she is still a child who needs the loving, pampering and attention of his parents. The child is still unable to understand why his mother or father is not spending so much time with him any more.

- The parents should not expect the child to be independent before he is ready for it. Often, parents expect the older child to suddenly grow up, become independent and do not give him time to learn gradually.
- The child's attempts to adjust must be acknowledged and appreciated.
- Both parents must make sure that they spend quality time with the child. This must be exclusive time, undisturbed by the baby. Parents can take turns in doing this.

CASE STUDY

This case study is from my own family. My first-born was an only child for 10 long years before the second one decided to come (due to my first one's prayers, as claimed by her). We had many fears regarding the future as we were not so young anymore and were not really prepared for this not-so-small surprise. Moreover, there would be a large age gap between our two children. Nevertheless, after much soul-searching and net surfing, we came to the conclusion that it was not the age gap that mattered; it was the quality of relationship that truly mattered. Many people we spoke to said that siblings who are much older double up as mini-moms and dads for their younger siblings. This reassured us and we decided to welcome the new arrival with a positive attitude. After the initial excitement, reality began to dawn. The jealousy and possessiveness that the older sibling normally feels when a new baby arrives were in evidence. As the baby started to grow and intrude into the personal space of the now pre-teen older sister, real trouble started brewing. As she grew even more, it became more and more like any normal sibling relationship. The usual 'She started it!' 'I did not! She started first!'... My husband and I were left wondering where was the 'mini-mother' we had been told to expect!

We soon began to realize that regardless of the age gap, siblings will be siblings and there was bound to be a rivalry. But my mother-in-law reassured me when she said, 'Boys will be friendly when young but fight when older, and girls will fight when younger but be friends for life.' I could now hope that my daughters would enjoy this eternal sisterhood, such as the one I now share with my own sister after years of fighting.

During the early years, when the foundations of the personality pattern are being laid, parents must divide their attention equally, or else the children may feel unloved and rejected. This can happen even at the tender age of 1 year, when emotions are formed, but not the ability to express them. The emotions get stored in their pre-conscious and the resentments can show up as destructive behaviour when they are adults.

Parents take it for granted that the child will adjust and adapt to the new circumstances, but these coping mechanisms may or may not be healthy for his future adjustment. The child's problem may exist for many years without the parents becoming aware of it. It is only when the child's mind begins to mature, between 12 and 20 years of age, that the hatred and fury which were bottled up inside over so many years begin to manifest as destructive behaviour against himself or others. By this time, it is much more difficult to find solutions to the problem.

There have been extreme cases where rapists and abusers have traced their problems back to their childhood, when their parents played favourites, and the subjects ended up generalizing their negative attitudes towards their mother or sister to all women.

How parents make it worse for siblings

Favouritism and clash of personalities

Generally, there is more talk of how parents influence the child's growth and development than what children bring into the relationship (nurture versus nature), i.e. their inborn personality traits. Each child is born with a different temperament. Some children are easy-going, do not trouble their parents for anything, do not cry at night and never have feeding problems. Then there are babies who are difficult right from birth—they cry excessively, want to be carried all the time and are very temperamental.

Parents are influenced by their children, even to the extent that their personalities may change after the birth of their children. A man who would never tolerate mediocrity from his colleagues finds himself becoming extremely patient after the birth of the first child. A woman who was known for her calm and composed nature might find herself screaming for the most trivial reasons while her child is growing.

According to Dr Rabie Azoory, a psychologist focusing on families, 'Children divide into divergent personality types, and the child who is more compliant and easy-going is the favoured one, because adults tend to like those characteristics better, and the one who is more angry, anxious and depressed is the disfavoured child. *And it is not easy for parents to accept this.* The theory goes that if there are two siblings born next to each other, they immediately develop opposing or divergent personality types. You will see that in any siblings who are born first and second. It is not about the birth order because the first-born may be either favoured or disfavoured. And, equally, the second born may be either favoured or disfavoured'.[23]

There may be no problem as long as children are unaware of whether they are favoured or disfavoured. But the parents may reveal these feelings in a fit of anger, and this leads to or reinforces sibling rivalry. Children may purposely act in the opposite way to the favoured child to establish their own identity. They may even try to overcompensate for their guilt about not liking the child by giving him excess love and affection.

How do parents overcome favouritism?

To this, Dr Azoory says: 'You really have to dig into your own feelings for that. The reason why I called it favouritism—many people reject that nomenclature, but it is favouritism because we fall into the pattern of favouring one child over the other. *You have to work with your feelings first* and make yourself feel as much for your disfavoured child as you do for the favoured one. And recognize that the disfavoured child's gripe and difficulty is dealing with his or her feeling of being a failure, or of holding a lesser position and status with the prime parent than the favoured child. So that is the crux of their pain, and when you address that pain by giving them respect and attention on the same level as you give to the favoured child, you heal and soothe them and they come around better. So, you really have to work with yourself. It is not an easy task. But they do come around, and when they come around, you gain more leverage because they begin to love you better and behave better.'

According to psychotherapists, nothing can be done about the situation until the parents, or anybody for that matter, accept that something is wrong and want to change the situation. Nothing can be done as long as the parents are in denial of their own feelings. But once they accept their own feelings (no matter how unacceptable they may sound to themselves), they will start noticing the changes immediately.

Comparison

Other than favouritism, this is one more way in which parents make matters worse.

The comparison between two children starts even before the birth of the second child, that is, during pregnancy. The mother may say, 'Oh, I never had it so hard the first time. I never had any vomiting. Now my nausea has no end. I'm bedridden and I don't know what more troubles I'm in for.' Or, 'This fellow is really giving me a hard time... right from pregnancy. Now he doesn't let me sleep a wink. My first one was such a breeze.'

A mother might tell the doctor, 'My first one doesn't eat at all, and my second one eats too much. What do I do?' Such thoughts occur due to the misconception of parents that all children should be the same. Many parents are unaware that there will be individual differences, even between twins, and they should gracefully accept these differences. Very often, it is the unrealistic expectations on the part of the parents that make life miserable both for themselves and their children.

Parents or would-be parents have to be prepared for the fact that each of their children will come with his or her own temperament. In rearing and educating their children, they have to be prepared to work with each particular child's innate temperament. What is important for the development of a child as a true human being is not the child's temperament, but his character. Character is the result of the child's innate temperament plus the child-rearing practices of the parents.

Sometimes, parents compare in spite of themselves, almost as a last resort when everything else fails, with the intention that the anger that comparison induces may actually goad the child into doing what he is expected to do. But very often we are not conscious of our actions and their consequences. Favouritism and comparison have effects that can last forever, leading to low self-esteem and feelings of inadequacy.

According to Adele Faber and Elaine Mazlish, authors of the best-seller *Siblings Without Rivalry*,[24] 'Whenever I was tempted to compare one child to another, I would say to myself, "STOP! DON'T!" Whatever you want to tell this child can be said directly, without any reference to his brother. The key word is *describe*. Describe what you see. Or describe what you like. Or describe what you don't like. Or describe what needs to be done.

'Instead of comparing one child unfavourably to another ("*Why can't you hang up your clothes like your brother?*"), speak to the child only about the behaviour that displeases you.

'Describe what you see. "I see a brand new jacket on the floor."

OR

Describe what you feel. "That bothers me."

OR

Describe what needs to be done. "This jacket should be in the closet."

'The importing thing is to stick with the issue of this one child's behaviour. Nothing his brother is or isn't doing has anything to do with him.'

Birth order

When the first child is born, it is like a dream come true for many parents, who were eagerly looking forward to the new arrival. They lavish all their time and attention on the baby, take tons of photographs, organize a grand party for the baby's first birthday, and most of all, spend a lot of time playing with this new living, breathing toy, savouring his every move and milestone.

By the time the second child is born, they have been there, done that. There is no more anxiety, they know what to expect, and they make sure they do not repeat the mistakes they made with the first one. Of course, the last borns also enjoy the baby status for a long time and are a little more pampered than the first one, and in many cases are actually pampered by the first child! But on the downside, the second child gets only half the attention that the first child got. There is not so much joy and celebration as there was the first time, not that the parents are any less happy. A look at the family album may show fewer photographs of the second child.

The younger one learns everything faster as he has a role model. He does not have to bear the burden of setting an example. He does not have to assume leadership and take on responsibilities. As for first-borns, they tend to develop leadership skills and are usually high achievers because of parental pressures and a desire to win back parental approval. However, they are also insecure because they have been displaced by the younger siblings. In addition, they resent having more responsibilities than the younger ones.

Unfavourable associations—cultural aspects

In India, this subject takes on a whole new dimension. It sometimes so happens that a family which has been just getting by in society is suddenly hit by lady luck—money, a new house, a car, profit at business—coinciding with the birth of the second child. This child then becomes the favourite and the favoured one.

If it is the kind of family that prefers boys and the second or third child is a boy, it goes without saying that this boy will have the last word in the family. In India, where female infanticide is still a reality, many parents from lower socioeconomic strata do not believe in educating the girl child. They consider it a waste of their money as the girl will be going away after marriage anyway. In smaller towns and in conservative urban families, girls are expected to chip in with the housework, while the boys are not expected to lift a spoon. This can lead to resentment and rivalries.

(Of course in modern well-placed Indian families, leave alone the girl child, nobody does any work; there are maids and helpers to do all chores.)

Favourable approaches

- *Decision-making.* We need to involve the older child in decision-making, especially when the new baby is born. You can consult the first child about whether the yellow cradle or the blue cradle looks better. This will help him to feel a part of the new development and make him feel important.
- *Joint experiences.* Parents need to make sure that the entire family shares joint experiences once in a while, when there is no competitiveness but a feeling that everyone is a winner when they all do something together.
- *Encourage communication of feelings.* The mistake parents make most often is negating the child's feelings. If a child says, 'I did not ask for a brother, take him away!' the most expected answer would be, 'How could you say that? He is your little brother!' But saying that is not going to make the child's feeling go away. The child can come to terms only if the parents accept that he is feeling what he is feeling. We should not judge the child's feelings; instead, we should try to understand where these feelings are coming from.

The mother of the child mentioned above had fortunately read the book *How to talk so children listen and listen so children will talk,*[25] She said, 'It seems to me, Paul, you have two feelings about the baby. Sometimes you're glad you have a brother. He's nice to play with. And sometimes you don't like having him at all! You just wish he'd go away.' Paul liked that. And once a week, he would tell his mother, 'Tell me about my two feelings, mommy.'

To many parents, responding in this manner may seem contrived and artificial. This is because they are not used to it. But once they start practising and see the benefits of correct responding, it will become second nature to them.

- *Gap between two children.* The parents should plan to allow sufficient time between the births of each of their children so as to try to avoid having more than one child needing the same kind of care and attention at the same time. Also, as mentioned earlier, if the older child is still very young, he or she will not yet have the capacity to understand the parents' explanations with respect to the efforts needed for the care of the new baby, but will tend to respond in a purely emotional, negative way. According to research, the ideal gap seems to be 3, or at the most 4 years, for they have to be close enough to be able to bond with each other when they grow up, too.
- *Protected time.* Parents need to spend time with each one of their children. They need to take the time to play an active part in shaping their child's mind, to share their life experiences with him, and to become a friend to him.
- When spending time with one child, do not talk about the other.
- Don't lock the children into their position in the family constellation (oldest, youngest, middle). Allow each child the opportunity to experience some of the privileges and responsibilities of the other.
- *Let each child know what it is about him that his siblings like or admire.* Just knowing about a sibling's positive feelings can make for a dramatic shift in a relationship.
- *Schedule family meetings.* We would not expect our cars to run

without periodic re-fuelling and maintenance, yet we expect our family unit to run without regular check-ups.

We need to deal with our own feelings, help our children to deal with their feelings, and somehow take all the raw, angry, confusing emotions generated by sibling rivalry and use them. Yes, use them to help siblings grow into more sensitive, aware, caring human beings. Use them to learn how to live together despite deep differences.

'The family is where we learn our relationship skills. And the way we relate to our children and teach them to relate to each other, even in the heat of battle, can be our permanent gift to them', say Adele and Elaine while concluding the summary of their book.

{ Section IV }

DEVELOPMENTAL ISSUES

{ Chapter 8 }

On Learning

The art of teaching is the art of assisting discovery.

—MARK VAN DOREN

I have never let my schooling interfere with my education.

—MARK TWAIN

What is learning?

Learning is a continuous process that begins at conception and ends at death. 'I am learning all the time. The tombstone will be my diploma', according to Eartha Kitt.

In *General Psychology* by Atkinson and Hilgard, learning is defined thus: 'Learning is a relatively permanent change in behaviour that occurs as a result of a prior experience.'[26]

According to Mark Smith, 'Not surprisingly, many theorists have been less concerned with overt behaviour but with changes in the ways in which people "understand, or experience, or conceptualize the world around them".[27] The focus for them is on gaining knowledge or ability through the use of experience.'

The depth or nature of the changes involved is likely to be different. In 1979, Säljö carried out a simple, but very useful piece of research. He asked a number of adult students what they understood by learning. Their responses fell into five main categories:

1. Learning as a quantitative increase in knowledge: Learning is acquiring information or 'knowing a lot'.
2. Learning as memorizing: Learning is storing information that can be reproduced.

3. Learning as acquiring facts, skills, and methods that can be retained and used as necessary.
4. Learning as making sense or abstracting meaning: Learning involves relating parts of the subject matter to each other and to the real world.
5. Learning as interpreting and understanding reality in a different way: Learning involves comprehending the world by reinterpreting knowledge.[28]

As Paul Ramsden comments, 'We can see immediately that conceptions 4 and 5 are qualitatively different from the first three. Conceptions 1 to 3 imply a less complex view of learning. Learning is something external to the learner. It may even be something that just happens or is done to you by teachers (as in conception 1). In a way, learning becomes a bit like shopping. People go out and buy knowledge—it becomes their possession. The last two conceptions look to the "internal" or personal aspect of learning. Learning is seen as something that you do in order to understand the real world.'[29]

Every animal and human is a natural learner. Learning is a natural and continuous process. A (relatively permanent) change in behaviour constitutes real learning. That is, when the learning is internalized or when it becomes a part of who we are.

Take the traffic rules. People wear helmets when there are fines imposed for not wearing them; people stop at red lights when there is a traffic policeman in sight. Once the rule is lifted or if there is no one watching, the rule is flouted. Why? Because the reason why the rule exists in the first place has not been learnt or internalized. The person in question has not understood why such a rule exists.

However, if one has met with an accident or witnessed an accident due to failure to follow the rule, the learning is internalized as the learning is accompanied by a real experience; the person may wear a helmet even if it is not compulsory any more, and may stop at a red light even at midnight!

How does learning take place?

What does this example demonstrate? For real learning to take place, it has to be experiential. It has to happen in such a way that the learner can relate to what he needs to learn. It has to be connected with his real-life experience. Else, it never enters the long-term memory, never gets internalized and never causes a change in the learner.

Take another example. I once asked a teacher of mine at school if she had child psychology in her BEd course (I cannot believe I actually had the nerve to ask her, for she was a terror to us!). She said yes, but that the trainees would never bother with it much as it was enough if they passed in the subject. What a sad state of affairs! I used to be her favourite one to pick on. Thanks to the self-esteem that my parents had managed to instil in me during my childhood years, I survived the ordeal and even came out shining. But think of those children who were not as lucky. Her not taking child psychology seriously left a gap in her education. The point is that if the teacher who taught the trainees child psychology had inspired them and had managed to connect the subject with their lives as children, they would then probably have studied it with interest and even taught their children with interest and inspiration.

Learning styles

The process of learning involves not only *knowing what* but also *knowing how*. In other words, it is not just the content which is imparted, but how it is imparted that is of the utmost importance if we really want students to learn something (*see* Box on pp 94–5).

In this context, my favourite analogy is that of my cleaning woman. What is her job? To clean. What is the tool that she uses? A broom. If I still see dirt left on the floor and question her about it, she says that she did sweep the floor. I ask her that she did sweep, but has she really 'cleaned', which is her primary goal? This is what happens in most schools when it comes to teaching. The teachers feel they have

Orientations to learning

Four orientations to learning (after Merriam and Caffarella 1991: 138)

Fifth added by Nirupama Rao about Steiner's Waldorf Education/Anthroposophy

Aspect	Behaviourist	Cognitivist
Learning theorists	Thorndike, Pavlov, Watson, Guthrie, Hull, Tolman, Skinner	Koffka, Kohler, Lewin, Piaget, Ausubel, Bruner, Gagne
View of the learning process	Change in behaviour	Internal mental process (including insight, information processing, memory, perception)
Locus of learning	Stimuli in external environment	Internal cognitive structuring
Purpose in education	Produces behavioural change in desired direction	Develops capacity and skills to learn better
Educator's role	Arranges environment to elicit desired response	Structures content of learning activity
Manifestations in adult learning	Behavioural objectives Competency-based education Skill development and training	Cognitive development Intelligence, learning and memory as function of age Learning how to learn
Anticipated outcomes		

Adapted from Smith MK. *'Learning theory', The Encyclopedia of Informal Education.* 1999, 2003.

Humanist	Social and situational	Spiritual
Maslow, Rogers	Bandura, Lave and Wenger, Salomon	Rudolf Steiner, J. Krishnamurthy, Montessori
A personal act to fulfil potential	Interaction/observation in social contexts. Movement from the periphery to the centre of a community of practice	0–7: Imitation 7–14: Imagination 14–21: Inspiration
Affective and cognitive needs	Learning is in relationship between people and environment	Understanding of the true nature of the human being and developmental needs of children at a given age
Becomes self-actualized, autonomous	Full participation in communities of practice and utilization of resources	Develops Individuality, realizes actual potential, develops complete human being
Facilitates development of the whole person	Works to establish communities of practice in which conversation and participation can occur	To serve as good role models, loving authority and partners and facilitators in the learning process
Andragogy Self-directed learning	Socialization Social participation Associationalism Conversation	Self-directed learning; holistic learning to balance thinking, feeling, willing; intuitive/meditative learning; encourage questioning and wait for answers; self-awareness and development
		Balanced temperament and personality, confident, compassionate, free thinking, initiative, responsible and contribute to society

www.infed.org/biblio/b-learn.htm.

done their 'job of teaching', which may involve reading the text out loud and then explaining it briefly and perfunctorily. She/he is in no way concerned if the students have learnt or not. But shouldn't that be the main concern of every teacher? We were taught in our course in Special Education that if a child is unable to learn the way you teach, you need to teach in a way that he can learn. This is a basic truth about the learning process that is not paid any attention to by schools.

As we have seen in the above illustration, if true learning has to take place, the subject has to be integrated into the child's experience. An effective way of doing this is by engaging the senses of the children—the senses of *touch, vision, hearing* and *movement.*

Parents and teachers need to realize that each one of us learns differently and through the senses. This is a scary thought for teachers, but it is now an established fact that different children learn differently.

Just recall the days when you were a student and you were preparing for an examination. How did you learn best? By reading aloud? By teaching an imaginary person? By writing on a board or notebook? By reading silently? Or by pacing up and down the terrace? Each one of us has a dominant sense that aids us in learning.

What happens in our schools is that teachers use only two senses to teach—visual, i.e. writing on the board, and auditory, i.e. explaining the lesson. So those children who have vision or hearing as their primary learning modality or sense learn very well. But what about those whose modality is touch or movement? They simply get left behind. They do not understand the lesson fully. And the saddest part is that they are blamed for not paying attention and for not scoring marks.

Progressive and alternative schools that have understood this have started incorporating all the four senses while teaching their lessons, by way of hands-on learning, such as projects, experiments, field trips, movement, art, music and so on.

Several schools in the modern era boast of the use of computers.

Using computers to learn is not the same as having a real experience out there in the world. A child cannot feel the roughness of a tree bark or smell the fragrance of a flower through a computer. Computers can never replace real sensory experiences. A child who has not experienced the world through his or her senses cannot be expected to understand the real world. A newspaper report about the children of Silicon Valley professionals stated that the children are being sent to a Waldorf school where they learn through real-life experiences and are kept away from computers.[30]

Unfortunately, when we talk about this in teacher training workshops, the most common response we get is, 'How do we do it when there are 60–70 children per class? It's simply not practical!' In reality, if the teachers are trained in such a way that they feel passionate about teaching, want to be facilitators rather than teachers, and want their children to love learning and to remember their lessons forever, this is the only way. Real-life experiences are being used very successfully in many schools across the world.

Learning in the context of education

If we are even remotely interested in the topic of learning, it is probably due to our concern about our children's education. Is it not true that as parents we are more interested in the marks our children get than in what they really learn at school?

Narayan Murthy, retired CEO of Infosys, has lamented the deterioration of the quality of students at IITs. This was bound to happen because we Indians are great when it comes to cracking competition, be it beauty pageants, the civil services or IIT. We are great at coaching students on a mass scale, teaching them to learn what is really important in terms of helping them pass the examinations. We are great at memorizing and reproducing. But what happens when our students enter the hallowed portals of the IITs? More memorizing and more reproducing. Our students are unable to come up with anything original any more! So where is the learning?

When we talk about learning, we need to talk about it at a very deep level. Learning is not memorizing. Learning is not passing examinations. Learning is something that changes lives. My teacher never learnt child psychology, but she cleared the paper. Her learning did not help her students learn.

Dear parents, what is it that we want for our children? Do we want our children to really learn something so that they can grow up to be complete human beings, or do we want them to just pass those examinations and get a great job?

I still remember, when I was a child, my father looked at my pathetic report card and then at my head hanging down in shame and asked, 'But tell me, did you learn anything new at school this term?' Would something like this happen in today's competition ridden times? All parents are afraid... afraid that their child will fall back and other children will race ahead if they do not push their child. They believe it is their duty as parents to push the child, even if they do not like the idea of pushing. If they do not push, they feel they may fail in their duty as parents.

Need for a balanced and holistic approach

Children are pushed to the limit; this is not an exaggeration. There have been numerous reports on the number of suicides in the IITs. Why? Every parent aspires that his child should go to an IIT. Whether the child is interested or not, whether he has the aptitude for engineering or not, that is the only way. The child is brainwashed into qualifying for the IIT from the elementary grade onwards. The emphasis is only on academics and marks and nothing else. Many children do manage to get into the IITs, but some fail in life.

Do we achieve the goal of education once the child is in IIT or IIM? Do we realize that along with academic skills it is also necessary to impart life skills to our children? Our children not only need to get great jobs; they also need to learn what it takes to be happy and complete human beings. Who is going to teach them these things?

The true purpose of education

This brings us to the true purpose of education. Why do we educate our children? What is the true purpose of education? Let us look at what some of the visionaries in education have said.

'Holistic education attempts to nurture the development of the whole person—this includes the intellectual, emotional, physical, social, aesthetic and spiritual.'[31]

Orr has said that 'the aim of holistic teaching is to facilitate a more fully integrated learning experience rather than the fractured and alienated learning experience and consequent life experience produced by much modern western pedagogy.[32]

Educational thinkers the world over have stressed the necessity of gearing education to the whole child. 'This thinking tends to be outside of the mainstream of educational thinking. Yet looking at the whole of a child's life is necessary when education is being used as a tool of transformation, empowerment and change', says Nancy Meaker in *A New Global Education*.[33] She adds: 'Intentionality behind how and why we are educating is extremely important. We must shift our perspective on education to the biggest picture and rethink the purpose behind education. Are we educating people to simply have skills and secure a job? Are we educating people so they know how to make the most of the land they live on? And ultimately, are we educating people on how to live a happy and fulfilling life, no matter what their circumstances?'

The noted thinker J. Krishnamurti asks, 'Now, what is the significance of life? What are we living and struggling for? If we are being educated merely to achieve distinction, to get a better job, to be more efficient, to have a wider domination over others, then our lives will be shallow and empty.... Though there is a higher and wider significance to life, of what value is our education if we never discover it? We may be highly educated, but if we are without deep integration of thought and feeling, our lives are incomplete, contradictory and torn with many fears; as long as education does not cultivate an integrated outlook on life, it has very little significance.... Education is not merely a matter of training the mind. A mind that has merely been trained is the continuation of the past, and such a mind can never discover the new. That is why, to find out what is right education, we will have to inquire into the whole significance of living.'

According to Rudolf Steiner, 'Our highest endeavour must be to develop individuals who are able out of their own initiative to impart purpose and direction to their lives.'[34] We need to remember that every human being has come into this world with a unique purpose. Parents do not realize that not every child is born to become an engineer. Many young software professionals and engineers have given up well-paying jobs to work for a cause that is close to their hearts, and money is not the most important thing for them.

Mahatma Gandhi said that 'the real difficulty is that people have no idea of what education truly is. We assess the value of education in the same manner as we assess the value of land or of shares in the stock-exchange market. We want to provide only such education as would enable the student to earn more. We hardly give any thought to the improvement of the character of the educated. The girls, we say, do not have to earn; so why should they be educated? As long as such ideas persist there is no hope of our ever knowing the true value of education.'

The real purpose of education, hence, is to bring up individuals who can think independently, who are compassionate and who can use their full potential to make this world a better place. Steiner says that a human being is made up of three aspects, namely, the head (intellect), the heart (compassion) and the hands (human will). If a human being is to be educated holistically, all three of these aspects need to be developed.

Sadhu Vaswani says that man has advanced so much technologically that he has reached the moon. But why is there so much unrest, violence and aggression in the world? That is because the heart is not developing at the same pace as the intellect.

A human being is much more than just intellect. According to the Dalai Lama, 'Everyone can understand that being human, we want to lead a happy life, to have a happy family, to be happy within ourselves. But material things alone will not provide us with genuine inner peace or inner happiness. Positive human values are essential. Just as parents bring up their children with love and care, teachers and school administrators need to make every effort to inculcate students with ethical values so that they grow up to be good human beings, with sound moral character and a commitment to the well-being of society. Passing examinations is not the be-all and end-all of education. Rather, we should bring up children in such a way that they grow up to be responsible individuals. *What is important here is what I call basic spirituality—the basic human qualities of goodness, kindness, compassion and care.* Whether we have religious faith or not, this kind of spirituality is essential. Without it, human existence remains something hard and dry. As a result, it is difficult to be happy. Our families, and ultimately society, will be more troubled. So, it is clear that cultivating these basic spiritual values is crucial to our well-being as a whole.'

Teaching the head, the heart and the hands

In the Waldorf schools, art is a major tool of teaching children in the elementary classes. Children are taught according to their developmental needs, and the curriculum is also designed to meet the physical, psychological and spiritual needs of the child. Steiner says, 'If one teaches things in a way that makes a one-sided claim on the child's intellect and the merely abstract acquisition of skills, then the development of the native will and sensibilities is checked; while if the child learns in a manner that calls upon its whole being, he or she develops all round. Drawing in a childish fashion, or even a primitive kind of painting, brings out the whole human being's interest in what he is doing. Therefore, one should let writing grow out of drawing. Beginning with an activity that, being artistic, draws out the whole human being, one should develop writing, which tends

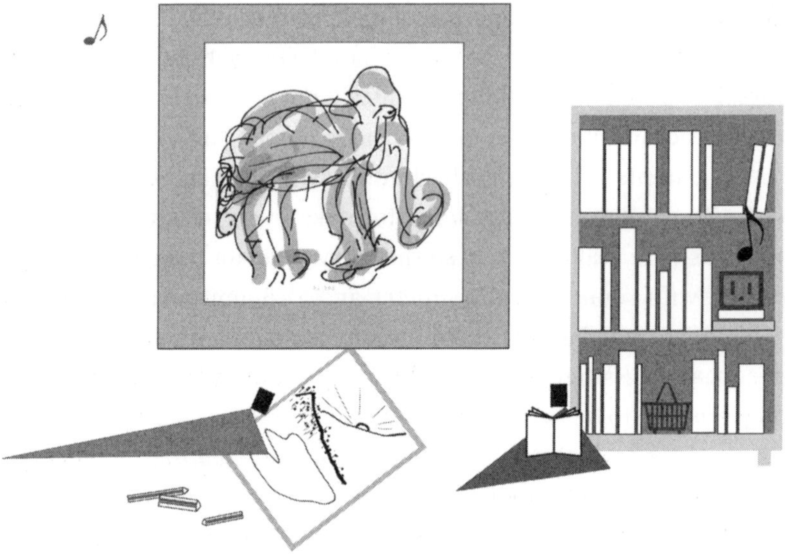

toward the intellectual. And one must let reading, which concentrates the attention strongly within the realm of the intellect, arise out of writing.'

Educating children by using art, music, movement and imagery gives rise to a 'life of feeling' in the children whence they are able to care for others and develop compassion and empathy (which is seriously lacking in our society today), while at the same time, helping them to engage more meaningfully with the lesson that is being taught. This calls for conscious effort, creativity and passion in the teacher. Imagine the impact of such an education on our society, if it could be imparted on a large scale—the instances of corruption, terrorism and crime could be drastically reduced.

'If the teacher engages his or her whole being in teaching, then he may safely bring the child things for which the full understanding will come when joyfully remembered in later life. There is something that constantly refreshes and strengthens the inner substance of life in this recollection. If the teacher assists such a strengthening, he will give the child a priceless treasure to take along on life's road', says Rudolf Steiner.[34]

Factors affecting learning

Teacher's attitude

Teachers have influenced our love and even our hatred for certain subjects just by the way they approach their job. Once again, according to Steiner, 'You have no idea how unimportant is all that the teacher says or does not say on the surface, and how important what he himself is as a teacher.'

This is important not just for teachers but also for parents, who should remember that the home is the first university and that parents are the child's first teachers. As human beings, we are often not conscious of our actions. We do not realize that children are watching us and learn by imitating us, especially until the age of seven or eight. We reprimand them for lying even though we lie blatantly in front of them while on the phone with the boss. Children easily catch on when we use double standards and do not hesitate to pull us up for them, that too, at the most inopportune moments.

Emotional well-being

Learning will take place at the optimal level when the child's emotional health is sound. For instance, the emotional climate at home, the marital relationship between the parents, the mental health of the parents, discord between various members of the family, etc. can affect the child's performance at school. To a certain extent, problems, disagreements and fights are common in every family, and most children are able to cope with the situation. But if the tension gets to a point where the child's needs for attachment, security and safety are not met, the lack of a healthy emotional climate at home will take its toll not only on the child's behaviour, but also on his academic performance, as his attention and concentration are affected. Therefore, if a child's grades are dropping, it may be worthwhile to examine what could be troubling him before actually reprimanding him for underperforming.

Learning disability

Ten to fifteen per cent of schoolchildren have a specific learning disability (SLD), a neurological condition that causes problems in reading, writing, spelling or arithmetic, which prevents optimum learning in spite of the child having average or above average intelligence. If the SLD is undiagnosed, the child is unjustly blamed or punished for a condition for which he or she is not responsible. Other than being of average or above average intelligence, a child with SLD sometimes possesses skills that children without SLD do not possess. *In learning, there can never be a disability, for these children just learn differently.* Their faculties include right-brain thinking, creativity and the ability to look at things from a different perspective. In fact, people with SLD who have been lucky enough to have supportive parents or teachers have gone on to become great achievers, using their special gifts. One has only to think of the success stories of Einstein, Edison, Leonardo da Vinci and Tom Cruise, who are some of the popular people diagnosed with SLD. Children with SLD can realize their potential only if they are taught in a specific, tailor-made and structured manner by specially trained teachers.

Recognizing that there is no such thing as a non-learner

All people are learners. The challenge is to determine the kind, amount and pace of learning that benefits different individuals, whether they are intellectually, developmentally or physically challenged. Every person loves to learn and wants to learn, but with dignity and freedom.

Encouraging and supporting the self-management of learning

Learners should be allowed to set their own goals and choose how and when to learn to meet needs that are identified by themselves

Learning is not just what happens in school. It happens all the time.

- Keep watching your children and keep giving them opportunities to learn by themselves. Do not solve their problems for them (as you may often be tempted to do) and rob them of an opportunity to struggle and hence to learn.
- Give them space to explore and grow. Do not overprotect them.
- The best learning takes place when it is spontaneous, joyful, self-motivated and, most importantly, when it happens in a non-threatening way in the total absence of anxiety.
- Do not give instant answers to all their innocent questions. Keep the childlike wonder alive by giving them magical answers. They will find the scientific answers on their own soon enough. It is important to retain the childlike innocence for as long as possible. Our children are growing up too fast. Let us allow them the time and space to be children a little longer.
- Do not fill their days with meaningless structured classes which kill their natural creativity.
- Children have a natural curiosity, a scientific bent of mind and a love for learning. Let us try to keep that alive in whatever way we can.

rather than others. An example of how this can be done is the use of programmed learning, in which learning is self-monitored. The theory of multiple intelligences by Howard Gardner and the principles of learning modalities are used to plan concept teaching, according to which children use one or more of their learning modalities (auditory, visual, tactile or movement) for testing out their concepts. Some schools even conduct open-book examinations—after the children are taught a lesson, they are sent off to the library to frame their own questions and find their own answers.

What examinations do is just to ensure that the student has 'studied the portions' for the examinations. The better one is at rote learning, the better his marks will be. But if one asks what the student has learnt, it may be difficult to answer, for we do not know if real learning has taken place.

We conclude this topic with words from *How Children Learn* by John Holt: 'Let me sum up what I've been trying to say about the natural learning style of young children. The child is curious. He wants to make sense out of things, find out how things work, gain competence and control over himself and his environment, do what he can see other people doing. He is open, receptive and perceptive. He does not shut himself off from the strange, confused, complicated world around him. He observes it closely and sharply, tries to take it all in. He is experimental. He does not merely observe the world around him, but tastes it, touches it, hefts it, bends it, breaks it. To find out how reality works, he works on it. He is bold. He is not afraid of making mistakes. And he is patient. He can tolerate an extraordinary amount of uncertainty, confusion, ignorance and suspense. He does not have to have instant meaning in any new situation. He is willing and able to wait for meaning to come to him, even if it comes very slowly, which it usually does.'

{ Chapter 9 }

Self-Esteem

To be beautiful means to be yourself. You don't need to be accepted by others. You need to accept yourself.

—THICH NHAT HANH

What is self-esteem?

Self-esteem is how a person feels about himself—his overall judgement of himself and how much he likes who he is. Self-esteem is not noisy conceit, which is but whitewash to cover low self-esteem, but a quiet sense of self-respect and self-worth. *In fact, self-esteem is the mainspring that slates every child for success or failure as a human being.*

The importance of self-esteem cannot be over-emphasized. As parents, only we can help our child to develop a firm and whole-hearted belief in himself.

Strong self-respect is based on two main convictions: 'I am lovable' and 'I am worthwhile' (I can love and deserve to be loved; I am competent to handle myself

A Reminder

I am enough
Just me alone
With no one's approval
Only my own

I am complete
With no need for more
Containing within me
An infinite store

I am abundance
I am magic and light
I am creation
I am joy and delight

I am Source of it all
I am boundless, and yet
Being still human
Sometimes I forget.

—DAN COPPERSMITH

and my environment; I know I have something to offer others). Each child, though thoroughly unique, has the same psychological needs to feel lovable and worthy. Nor do these needs end with childhood. You and I have them, and they will be with us until we die.

Every normal infant is born with the potential for good psychological health. But whether that potential flourishes depends on the psychological climate he lives in. To know whether the climate surrounding your child nurtures or withers, you must understand:

- how self-esteem is built, and
- how a child's self-view affects his behaviour.

How self-esteem is built

Eric Berne, the father of transactional analysis (TA), postulated that people make decisions in childhood that shape the rest of their life 'script'.[35] The script theory hypothesizes that people can choose lifelong tragic scripts—such as suicide, murder or alcoholism—in childhood. These choices are supported by routinely recurring games and the roles that people habitually play in them.

People actually seek out or create circumstances which will confirm these faulty life scripts. This is the reason why many women with poor self-image time and again seek out men/partners who turn out to be abusive. They do so because they deeply believe that they deserve it. Many children who are abused are given the message that they are being abused because they are 'bad' or 'dirty'. Hence, they believe that they truly are so and seek out circumstances that are punitive and that fit their life script, and only then are they satisfied.

Studies have shown that self-esteem is not related to family wealth, education, geographical living area, social class, father's occupation, or always having one's mother at home. It comes instead from the quality of relationships that exist between the child and those who play a significant role in his life.

How many people out there actually believe they are good, worthy and adequate? People with low self-esteem far outnumber those with good self-esteem. There are reasons for this.

Positive strokes and negative strokes

We humans find it easier to recognize and acknowledge bad behaviour and the negative rather than good behaviour and the positive. We lose no time when we want to criticize somebody, but hold back when it comes to appreciating something even when it is truly deserved.

According to TA, when young children form their life scripts, they subconsciously count the number of positive strokes (appreciation) and negative strokes (criticism) that they receive from their environment. On the basis of whichever outweighs the other, they form an opinion about themselves and decide for life whether they are 'good enough' or 'bad enough'.

This is the reason why it is important for us to remember never to use the terms 'good boy' or 'bad boy' when we talk to children. Children take the term as a character judgement, include it in their life script and decide their opinion of themselves on its basis. Instead, we need to make sure we are clear which behaviour it is that we are approving of and which one we are not by specifying, 'That was bad throwing' or 'That was good sharing'.

There are no good/bad children, only good/bad behaviour. Even the bad behaviour occurs for a reason. No child wants to be bad. If he is indulging in bad behaviour, he is trying to communicate something through it. It could be that he is hungry, tired, sleepy or bored, or maybe he just needs you to pay attention to him.

The subtle and the unspoken messages

When children are very young, they develop much of their sense of self-worth by studying how others perceive them. These others include parents, other family members, school teachers, friends and other important people in the child's life. The messages that children receive from these significant others can be verbal, including through the tone of voice, and through attitudes, judgements and body language. Words have power. They can build or shred self-respect. But words must be matched by actions; unless they are, children can detect the discrepancy and this is more dangerous than direct negative words. Children then learn not to trust what we say. For example, a mother may say, 'I love you' to the child often, but is not physically present when the child needs her the most, or even when present, if she does not listen with full attention, the child will draw his own conclusions about her true feelings.

We all know for sure how perceptive children are. Parents are always surprised by how much children know and how they pick up information from adult conversation even when they seem to be busy playing. Apart from the fact that in the children's presence, we should refrain from talking about what we would not like them to hear, we also need to remember that children pick up what is unspoken as well.

One could never tire of repeating Rudolf Steiner's quote about how it is not so important what we say or do, but it is indeed important who we are. No matter what we say or how we act in the presence of our children, they know exactly *who we are.* They can see through our facade and form their scripts based on what they perceive under our skin. Scary thought, isn't it?

Perhaps this is the real secret behind the saying, 'The child is father of the Man.' We can learn from our children who we are and how to become a real human being if we are awake (conscious) enough. They are mirrors to our soul. I have heard moms tell me that when they see their daughter doing something unacceptable, they realize with utter disbelief that this is exactly what they do!

Unfortunately, our children are dependent on us and a lot depends on how awake we are when it comes to child-raising. Their self-esteem and feelings of adequacy depend not only on the strokes we give them, but as they learn through imitation, it also depends on our opinions about ourselves. Yes! Children also imbibe our attitudes, do

CASE STUDY

Once upon a time, there was a little boy called Dave. His mother was an alcoholic, a woman of unstable mind. He had other brothers, but he was the one his mother chose to abuse. He had to live in the basement, alone, without food, sometimes for days together. She would abuse him physically and torture him, and once even burnt his hands on the stove. Little Dave hoped to find someone who would love him and did find someone. But his childhood experiences led him to believe that he was not worthy of love. He would actually try to push away the person who came forward to love him. Fortunately for him, this person was persistent as she understood where the resistance was coming from. She was patient and she helped him to love himself. She helped him to understand that he was not responsible for what had happened to him. Slowly, he began to listen and he started to let love into his life.

Today, Dave Pelzer is a best-selling author (*A Child Called 'It', A Man Named Dave*), inspirational speaker and internationally renowned humanitarian, who travels throughout the world talking to and inspiring others whose self-esteem is bruised and who were also abused. His mission is to help them believe that no matter what happens to them on the outside, inside them shines a loving light that can illuminate the whole world.[36]

they not? If they see their mother standing in front of the mirror, they also see the look of either satisfaction or dissatisfaction on their mothers' faces. Body image is a totally learned behaviour.

Role of the media

The role of the media is of the utmost importance in this age of six-pack abs and size-zero figures. Undue importance is being given to body image. With television taking up large chunks of our waking time, and with commercial breaks being longer than the actual programme, we are constantly being bombarded with the messages of the commercials. The industry plays on people's emotions and takes unscrupulous advantage of the fact that we are always judging ourselves on the basis of the colour of our skin, the size of our waist and our height. Not a single body part is left out. Young, impressionable minds take these messages seriously and spend endless hours lamenting what they do not have.

Self-image is also influenced by the brands a person can show off and the gadgets he carries. Banks line up to give loans and credit cards to help us satisfy our endless cravings. An entire economy is thriving on the self-esteem issues of our population.

Children with a healthy self-image are not affected by what they see in the advertisements or what their friends are using. They may demand these things at one point or the other, but when the parents sit with them and explain the reason why they do not feel they should buy it, they can understand and accept it.

How a child's self-view affects him

It is believed that a child's self-concept colours his behaviour. Whenever a youngster sees himself as a loser, he expects to fail and behaves in a way that makes success less likely. On the other hand, a youngster with a history of past successes expects to do well.

Low self-esteem acts as a roadblock to personal happiness by preventing successful social involvements. If an individual has low self-worth, this will be reflected in his interpersonal relations, leading to greater dissatisfaction and increased feelings of inadequacy, thereby perpetuating the cycle.

Self-esteem and identity

Self-acceptance is the springboard for all our successes and failures.

Accepting oneself is a particularly difficult task for the adolescent. The familiar and comfortable self he has known in childhood is in a state of change. All the changes in his body (i.e. sexual development, physical size and muscular development) and changes in his cognitive development necessitate a modification of his childhood self. He is constantly told by others that he is growing up, and with this growth come new responsibilities, certain rights and advantages, and expected behaviour. Consequently, he begins to ask questions such as: 'Who am I?', 'What do I believe in?' and 'Would others like me if they knew what kind of person I am?'

Without a positive and strong sense of identity, many teenagers suffer from low self-esteem and self-doubt. Identity formation often involves making new friends, joining certain clubs or sports teams, getting involved with a youth group, beginning to separate emotionally from one's parents or enrolling in certain classes at school. Ideally, the teenager emerges from the process stronger and more confident, knowing who he is and thinking he knows what he wants out of life.

Self-esteem and well-being

Many youngsters (and adults) whose behaviour is detrimental to themselves and to society as whole—dropouts, delinquents, alcoholics and dope users—privately believe that they are hopelessly inadequate and worthless. Low self-esteem can also lead to poor relationships, anxieties, depression and even suicide.

When it comes to teenagers, it is important to find out their likes, interests and talents and encourage them. As Einstein said, 'Everybody is a genius. But if you judge a fish by its ability to climb a tree, it will spend its whole life believing that it is stupid.' Do not try to push a teenager into something that is beyond his ability and outside his area of interest. If teenagers are encouraged to work on their strengths, they will feel good about who they are and can realize their potential.

When children grow into adulthood with good self-esteem, they are better able to work constructively on the problems and inequities that exist in our world. Their solid cores free them to be innovators rather than destroyers, and they can contribute constructively to society.

What can be done to foster high self-esteem:

- Listen actively with focused attention. We need to be fully present and not be distracted even by our thoughts. This communicates to the child the message that, 'I love you so much that I am putting aside everything else in order to be with you.'
- Accept your child's feelings without being judgemental. They are important and need to be acknowledged. We need to know what children feel about various matters in order to know what they feel about themselves.
- Rather than using the terms 'bad boy' or 'bad girl', comment on the behaviour that is bad or good.
- Respect the differences among your children and plan actively for these, both in terms of your expectations and family activities.
- Your expectations are more likely to be fair if they are based on the facts of child development, alert observation and sensitivity to the past and present pressures on the child.
- The more fulfilled you are as a person, fewer will be the unrealistic pressures you will put on your child.
- Children who do not receive the right balance of discipline (clear and consistent limits) and love cannot grow up with high self-esteem. They tend to feel more dependent and also feel that they have less control over their world.

- Children will run into disapproval and cruelty in the world. They need the emotional protection of the parents' belief in them to grow their self-esteem and to face all odds. This applies to all human beings, whether or not they are handicapped or disabled.
- Democratic methods of discipline, which are based on mutual respect, realistic expectations, skill in releasing negative feelings and a willingness to share one's feelings and power, encourage responsibility, independence, motivation, creative thinking, intellectual growth, personal involvement and respect for those in authority. They directly enhance self-esteem, for they are powerful proofs of love, faith and trust.
- Ignore negative behaviour if it is not harmful to the child or others. Distract the child to focus on something else. Appreciate small gestures by giving the child an approving glance or a pat on the back, or ruffling his hair. One need not go overboard with praise either.
- Touch and warmth play a very important role in helping a child develop good self-esteem. Do not hesitate to hug him or physically demonstrate your love from time to time. Children need our touch and warmth. They thrive on it. It is a basic physiological need.

{ Chapter 10 }

Teaching Children Values

Integrity is doing the right thing even when no one is watching.

—OPRAH WINFREY, Talk show host

It is not difficult to make decisions when you know what your values are.

—ROY DISNEY, American film writer, producer, nephew of Walt Disney

Values are the ideas you have about what is important and what is not; what is good and what is bad; what is right and what is wrong. Values are something that you use as a standard for judging yourself and the rest of the world. You may never have stopped to think about your values. Nevertheless, they are there, standing behind your beliefs, attitudes, interests and goals. Values give meaning and direction to every part of your life, especially in the area of how you parent your children. *Values are at the core of our being—of who we are and what we do.*

It is actually fun to start to think of what you stand for, and to write your values down. Where do you stand on some of the following?[37]

- Honesty and integrity
- Kindness
- Sticking together as a family and supporting each other
- Fairness
- Taking into account each family member's feelings (both positive and negative)
- Cooperation and thoughtfulness

- Reliability
- Good manners
- Responsibility
- How to treat people worse off than you
- The importance of education
- Kindness to helpless animals
- Acceptable behaviour and consequences of certain actions
- How to respond to people more important/rich/famous than you
- How important each family member is
- Eating healthy food and looking after our bodies
- Respect for authority

Now rank the five most important values. These are the values that are crucial to you.

How children learn values

Experiences and relationships in the early years form the foundation of the system of values that a person has in later years. A warm, accepting love on the part of the parents helps nurture desirable attitudes and feelings. Children learn values in their growing-up years, but a complete value system is not developed until late adolescence.

Children learn about values in small doses, day in and day out.

Each of us has a unique value system, almost as unique as our fingerprints. A value system is not only passed down from parents or learnt through schools, etc. but is also fine-tuned and developed through personal experiences, in combination with the values that our immediate society (that is, the social circle in which we live and the people with whom we interact) lends to us. Take the example of a teenager who has learnt from her parents that taking drugs is harmful. Now this girl belongs or wants to belong to a popular group in her class. This group is a 'cool gang' and these children have to do 'cool' things like sniffing drugs. The choice that the teenager will make—whether to try drugs in order to belong or refuse as she has been taught—will depend on the values she has been taught, how she has been taught and how desperately she wants to belong.

Your values have a great effect on your children. But children also pick up other ideas about values from everything and everyone around them. Hence, we need to play an active role in learning about how children pick up values and helping them learn what is important.

Getting a good grounding

One often hears this description about a person, 'He's really grounded.' Where does this come from? There is an entire philosophy behind this. Values, ethics and morals are higher-order thinking. Taller buildings invariably need stronger, deeper foundations. We can give you two illustrations to make this clear.

According to Rudolf Steiner, there are not just the five physical senses, but there are 12 senses in all, as shown in the diagram below. The four lower senses help us get to know ourselves, the four middle

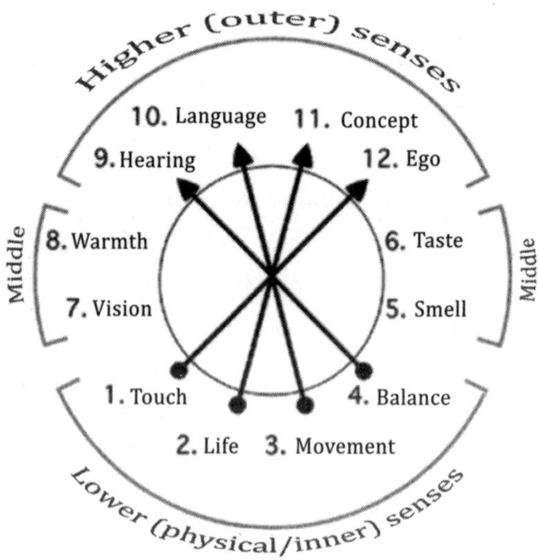

Rudolf Steiner's 12 senses
http://www.movementforchildhood.com/12senses.pdf

senses help us get to know the world around us, and the four higher senses help us to get to our higher selves and other human beings.

In order to develop the higher senses of understanding others, children need a good grounding in the lower senses in the early years, at least up to the age of 7 years. They need to be stimulated in these senses. For this we need to encourage them to explore the natural physical world with their hands, feet and in fact, their entire being. They need to use their hands and move a lot, and do plenty of balancing activities. We used to do all of this when we were kids, when there was still outdoor space to explore, trees to climb and walls to jump over. There was plenty of full-fledged physical play before television kidnapped our children.

As shown in the diagram, the lower senses are directly connected to the respective higher senses. Hence, children who get a good grounding and literally connect with the earth are able to develop higher-order thinking. The lower senses are the foundation of our existence. The book *The Best Days of My life,*[38] which describes the childhood of some of the world's greatest persons such as Einstein, Abraham Lincoln, Kapil Dev, Da Vinci and Marie Curie, illustrates the case in point. These people spent their childhood in the woods, mountains and countryside, bonding with and enjoying the beauty of nature, chopping wood, making shoes, farming and doing hard physical labour. It is this grounding that took them to the highest levels in life.

When one spends time with nature, one begins to respect it and gets to learn from the tiny creatures the value of respecting each other's space and not impinging on it without reason. Ironically, we human beings are the only creatures who are capable of higher order thinking, but behave worse than insects and animals.

A major factor that is detrimental to getting a good grounding is urbanization and changing lifestyles. Added to this is the emphasis on early intellectual and academic education. When we start academics too early, expose children to too much information too early through television, encyclopaedias and computers, the process of grounding gets affected and we see that the children are not calm and peaceful.

On the other hand, we find that children from small towns and those from families who know this truth are more in control, courteous, balanced, well-adjusted and mature (this is different from precocity, where the child has a lot of knowledge and displays adult-like behaviour which is not necessarily age-appropriate). These are the children who inherently possess good values—they value themselves and others. They show respect, consideration and responsibility towards others.

It is possible to work towards giving our children a good grounding if we try to understand the matter in a deeper way.

Even Abraham Maslow's hierarchy of needs refers to the same thing, i.e. the higher needs cannot be achieved unless the lower needs are taken care of (*see* the diagram below).

Hence, in order to develop good values, we need to have a

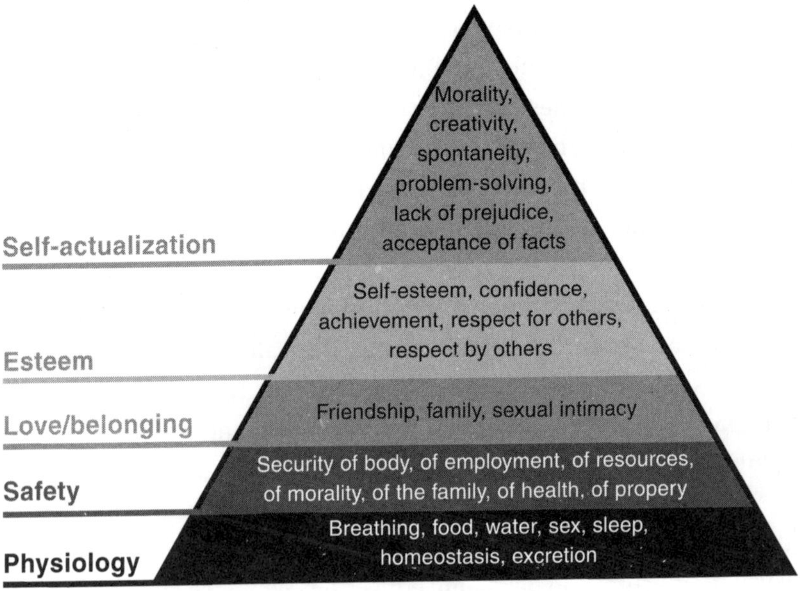

Maslow's hierarchy of needs
(http://psychology.wikia.com/wiki/Maslow's_hierarchy_of_needs)

CASE STUDY

I happened to witness this incident in the building where I live. This is a place where there are as many *didis* as there are children. There was this boy, about six or seven, who, together with his cycle, was being accompanied back from play by his *didi*. The *didi* looked very tired and was probably unwell. She could hardly walk. She was somehow lugging his cycle, waiting for the lift. She told him to please take charge of the cycle as she was very tired. He said that he would not. She requested him yet again. At this point, he lost his temper and threatened to complain to his mother that she was yelling at him. She kept quiet after that, maybe knowing that he could actually do that. One who witnesses this might think that the boy was rude and insensitive. But the thought that came to me was that probably he did not have good role models.

perspective that is guided by the heart and our intuition rather than an intellectual one guided by the mind.

Historical perspective

The world's great authors, poets, thinkers and philosophers have had the ability to impart value education to people in the simplest language, so that even the uneducated can understand the truths of life. Sant Kabir, Vemana, Vishnu Sharma, Aesop, Leo Tolstoy, Rabindranath Tagore and Ramakrishna Paramahamsa are some of the famous saints, poets and writers who have taught us about character and values in the simplest of language. Indian culture has handed down to its children the *Panchatantra, Jataka tales* and *Hitopadesha*, among other works of literature, which teach the important lessons of life through animal characters. These literary works, written many many years ago are still valued in our society. The reason is that no matter how much progress societies make, the basic human values remain the same.

Walking the talk

Some of the greatest philosophers, including Khalil Gibran and Rumi, the Sufi poets, Confucius, the Chinese Nobleman, and our own Mahatma Gandhi, Ramakrishna Paramahamsa and Tagore, taught values to generations of people not only through simple and captivating stories, poems and anecdotes, but also by walking the talk. They were living examples of what they preached. One of the stories I love telling about the integrity of the Mahatma is as follows.

One day, a woman went to meet Bapuji with a young child. She complained that the child was eating too much *gur* (jaggery) and said that the girl would stop if he would tell her to. Bapuji asked the woman to come back after a month. The woman was surprised, but was sure that he had a good enough reason for asking her to do this. She came back after a month and Bapuji told the little girl to stop eating *gur* as too much of it was not good for health. The woman could not help asking Bapuji why he needed a month's time to say such a simple thing. To this, Bapuji replied, 'This was not simple at all! A month back, I was eating a lot of *gur*... when I am doing something, how can I stop someone else from doing the same thing? This past month, I've been able to give up the habit myself, so now I'm in a position to tell her to stop.' Such was the integrity of the leaders who shaped the destiny of our country.

This kind of integrity is required of every parent and teacher if we have to teach children values. If children do not see adults doing what they are saying, they will never see why they should do it themselves. This is the eternal truth.

Is there a teacher from your school or college days whom you can never forget? Think about him or her for a moment. What is it about him or her that you remember and cherish?

- Was it the respect that he/she showed children even though they were years younger?
- Did he/she empathize with the children before blaming them for bad behaviour?
- Did he/she demonstrate such passion for the subject he/she taught that the students ended up loving it too?
- Was there congruence between his/her spoken word and unspoken body language?
- What were the values that he/she displayed?

There must be so many unsung heroes and leaders who are honest to their values and beliefs and who must be unconsciously shaping the lives of all the people they touch.

Present-day scenario

Indians living abroad are known to be sincere, hard-working and committed to work. However, our country is not the same as the one left behind by our great leaders. The values held by our culture (typical Indian values such as integrity, respect for elders, honesty, duty-mindedness and compassion) have, over many centuries, been eroding under the pressure of so-called modernization or westernization. While people in the West are looking to eastern philosophy and spirituality for peace, we, instead of learning from their mistakes, are blindly walking in the path laid out by them, refusing to see the consequences. The dissolution of joint families, absent parents, slavery to technology, breaking up of the family system, competition rather than cooperation, success at any cost—all these are resulting in a society stripped of its values.

What is missing?

There is more need today than ever before to consciously teach values to our children. As discussed in the section on the generation gap, in the past, learning of values was automatic and taken for granted.

In the days prior to television, the children's favourite pastime used to be to cuddle up to their grandmothers and ask them to tell them stories—either stories from their past or stories from mythology. Value education was an intrinsic part of these stories and thus, values were absorbed unconsciously and blended into the child's mind and soul.

But where are the grandmothers today? Where are the story sessions? Where are the value lessons? Even stay-at-home parents are using television as a babysitter and their energy resources seem to be drained out due to stress when it comes to telling bedtime stories. In fact, most parents must be dozing off halfway through a story even before the child falls asleep.

Talking about stories, an important aspect is that we tend to state the moral of the story after we tell it. There is an interesting and alternative perspective to this. Children absorb more when we do not state the moral we expect them to learn from it. For there may be more that a child gets from the story than what is specified. Leo Tolstoy never believed in stating the moral as it makes the story preachy and hence, less acceptable.

What can we expect our children to learn from babysitters, day-care centres, the television and computers? They learn about teenage romance, drugs, violence, hatred, indiscriminate killings and revenge—the themes of various television programmes, films and video games. Many older children belonging to the upper middle class have free access to the internet and there is hardly any supervision of the content they are being exposed to. There is a new ailment in this century—addiction to video games, Facebook, pornography, etc. for which de-addiction centres are opening in many countries.

Another affliction of the present generation is the spirit of competition, which has superseded the spirit of cooperation. It is a dog-eat-dog world and parents are pushing their children lest they get left behind. Children are encouraged to succeed at any cost and ethics are often compromised. The football coach and teacher since

23 years, Michael Koehler, has aptly said: 'In schools, we recognize and reward children for academics and athletics, but wouldn't it be great if there was an award for the kindest, most helpful, or most generous student?'[39]

Arise, awake!

So parents, the alarm bells are ringing and it is time to wake up and take stock of things. What do you want for your children? Do you want them to be super-achievers who score a zero on personal fulfilment and human values, or do you want them to lead a life of meaning and purpose? How do we find time in our busy lives to make sure that our children are growing up with the right values? The following are some important values and how we can inculcate them in our children.

Money talk

Parents these days complain that their children do not know the value of money, which is all the more worrisome in these times of big spending, shopping malls and multiplexes. How do children learn the value of money? Money is definitely more easily available today with the new economy, so they have everything even without asking. The parents would have grown up in a humble middle class family, in a small town in India, and budgeting and planning would have been a must before spending. But their children are born in big cities and they do not have to think much before they spend. The family eats out often, and the children are witness to budget-less grocery shopping and impulse buying. With these inputs, they do not really feel that there is a need to think before they buy something. They want it, so they should have it. If the mother ever says, 'Not now... I'm not carrying enough cash,' the child is ready with, 'So what? Use your credit card!'

- Parents should reflect on and examine the kind of example they are setting.
- They need to explain some of their buying decisions, e.g. why a particular product has more value for money and why one should go for discount sales.
- They should explain the difference between needs (running shoes), wants (branded shoes) and desires (branded shoes with special features such as lights or skates).
- They should ask themselves whether they are buying something their child really does not need.
- Parents often buy what they would have liked to have had as children.
- They should explain how credit cards and ATM cards work and that one is paying even if one cannot see it.
- Talking about the importance of budgeting would be useful. They should practise this themselves.
- Parents should talk about the importance of saving. Let the children start young with small amounts.
- The habit of giving to charity should be inculcated from an early age, with one portion of what the child gets going to charity.
- It is important to consciously avoid instant gratification. Our children need to learn to wait for something they need badly. The real and important things never come instantly.

Responsibility

Responsibility begins early in life with the parent–child bonding and with the child learning to value the time spent together with his parents. In the time they spend together with their children, parents can involve them in household chores such as dusting, watering plants, vacuuming and cooking (the child can be given his own miniature pretend tools). These chores should end up becoming an opportunity to have fun together, rather than a drudgery that needs to be got over with. The child feels a sense of accomplishment and feels proud that he is capable of doing something good.

Slowly graduate to giving your child minor jobs that are real and have value in the running of the household. Move from supervision to independence. This will go a long way in building the value (a character trait, in fact) of being reliable while doing a job.

Courage

At a young age, say at 3 or 4 years, children need the loving support of their parents to face their fears. Parents can talk to their children about their own fears and how they tried to overcome them, or how they are still trying to. This will enable the children to accept and overcome their own fears. An example will make this clear. Once a father pretended that he was afraid of the dark, to help his son. He held his son's hand and walked into a dark room, saying, 'I am calm and in control, I am calm and in control!' The son saw the father slowly feeling better. He eventually tried it himself and it really worked!

At an older age, children need courage to stand up to what they believe is the right thing to do. They require courage if they have to say no to something which they are pressurized to do, like trying a cigarette, shoplifting or even trying drugs.

Courage does not have to be loud and noisy. It can be a quiet but strong feeling that one is right; one knows it and is going to stick with it, even if it means rejection.

In the words of a 10-year-old child, 'Fearlessness is just foolish bravado. But courage is to face that which you fear most.'

Integrity

What is the difference between integrity, on the one hand, and values, morals and principles, on the other? Having values, morals and principles means to know what the right thing to do is, whereas having integrity is actually doing the right thing. How do we teach integrity?

When a child makes a mistake like lying or stealing, ask the child, 'When you were about to do this, was there a part of you that said, "Don't do it?"' There will be a meaningful pause as the child reflects upon the question. Most likely, he will say yes. Then you can say, 'But you did not listen to it, did you?' And add, 'Don't worry. You will get plenty more opportunities to listen to that voice. Listen to that little voice inside your head. It will always tell you what is the right thing to do.' And thus close the matter.

Conclusion

Teaching values cannot be limited to a single period once a week. There are umpteen opportunities in everyday life to teach children values. If parents are present in body, mind and soul, they can use various opportunities to teach their children important lessons about life. It could be in transit, for example, while in a car or train, while waiting in a line or while doing chores together.

No matter how much we try to teach them, children learn from who we are as human beings and most importantly from life itself. Experience is the best teacher and if the experience each time is the same it gets reinforced. They may not seem to do what we are currently doing by way of imitation, but when they leave the nest, it is these values that they have imbibed from us that will help and protect them and give them a sense of security to face challenges in life.

{ Section V }

SPECIAL ISSUES

{ Chapter 11 }

Adoption

I knew I loved my daughter from the first moment I found out she was growing inside me. Although I knew I was too naive, young and poor to raise her myself, there was never a question she would be brought into this world. I loved her father even though we would never see each other again; therefore, the only sensible choice was open adoption. I loved my child too much to hand her over to people that I had never met. My feeling was and always will be that if I was too scared to look these people in the face, to know and love and bond with them, then how in the world could I in good conscience hand my baby over to them never to see her again? I know without a second of guilt or remorse that I made the right choice in open adoption. How can there be a negative side? Now my child not only has one set of family members who love her, but 2, 3, 4.... How can it be bad to have more people love you rather than less? Now, when each of us wakes up each day to face a new part of our lives, there are no haunting, unanswered questions to get in the way of our feeling secure in who we are, so that we may face the rest of our challenges with that knowledge on our side. Now, I feel like I have a second family too, not just my daughter.

—JENNIFER BOUCHARD DOANE,
birth-mother and life-mother

I had not realized how adversely closed adoption and the absence of my biological history had affected me until I gave birth to my son Gabriel. When I held him in my arms, for the first time in my life I felt connected to the earth.

—Adoptee and adoptive parent CORI

> *There is no doubt in my mind that being adopted affects parenting in a profound way. But how it manifests itself is as idiosyncratic as each parent, as unique as each child.... We can only do our best to follow our hearts, to watch both ourselves and our children with a compassionate eye, and to find out our own place on the ever-lilting balance beam of parenthood.*
>
> —SUSAN ITO, Adopted child

> *Not flesh of my flesh, nor bone of my bone,*
> *But still miraculously my own.*
> *Never forget for a single minute,*
> *You didn't grow under my heart - but in it*
>
> —FLEUR CONKLING HEYLINGER

Adoption is not a new concept in this world. There have always been children without parents, parents without children, and parents and children who have found love when they found each other. Mythology and history abound with happy and some not so happy stories involving adoption. Moses, Krishna, Sita, Karna and Shakuntala were all adopted children. Moses was a Hebrew child adopted by an Egyptian queen. Krishna, who was born to Devaki, was adopted by Yashoda, and Yashoda's love of Krishna was the epitome of a mother's love. Sita was the gift of mother earth to King Janaka. Karna was born to the unwed mother, Kunti, and was brought up by a charioteer. He remained loyal to his adoptive parents even after he got to know about his parentage.

One of my students, a child with special needs and his older sister, were adopted by NRI parents. When they realized that life in the USA was not helping their son, they came to live in India for a year to seek therapy for him. They found that in terms of lifestyle, food, therapy and schooling, India had much more to offer their son, so they resettled in India. This is exemplary for any parent to do for his child. It is believed that a parent's love for his child goes beyond the biology of parenting.

Adoption has received added media coverage due to celebrity couples adopting children from developing countries; for example, film stars such as Madonna, Anjelina Jolie and Brad Pitt. Back home, Sushmita Sen has set the trend for single-parent adoption. With homosexuality being legalized in many countries, many gay couples are coming to India for surrogacy and adoption. India is, in fact, one of the favoured countries for couples looking to adopt.

Adoption is twice as wonderful as bringing up a biological child because it serves reciprocal purposes—it gives the child a loving home and it gives loving parents a wonderful child.

Secrecy about adoption

Although adoption is not new, the increasing openness about adoption is relatively new. Adoption is, to a great extent, still shrouded in a veil of secrecy. The reasons for this secrecy could be:

- The parents are anxious that the child may feel unhappy about not being his parents' biological child.
- The parents are also afraid that someone may make hurtful comments about the child's adoptive status.
- Not being able to produce a child can be looked upon with prejudice or pity in our society, as is often depicted in the films, so the parents may want to keep the adoption confidential.

Today many couples are opting not to have children as they are clear about what they want in life. However, the scenario differs when the couple is unable to have a baby. They may accept it, but from what I have seen among my friends, it is the elders of the family—the well-meaning aunts and other relatives—who keep enquiring about the family status, much to the discomfiture of the couple. But this is changing.

Changing scenario

Things are much different today than what they were, say, 20 years ago. There is more openness about adoption and in the matter of informing other people and one's own children about adoption.

According to Mrs Shanti of the Aashraya children's home, the age at which parents want to adopt has also been decreasing, especially in the past five to six years. Ten years back, parents who wanted to adopt were usually in their forties. Now people in their thirties are seeking to adopt children.

In the beginning, adoption used to take place within families to ensure a secure family background. Subsequently, couples used to ask for a child belonging to a specific religion or caste and so on, but of late, couples have not been asking for any specific trait of the child for adoption.

What motivates couples to adopt?

Childlessness is one of the main reasons for adoption. It is a condition that gives rise to a complex of emotions in the two individuals involved. They generally try out all the medical procedures before deciding to adopt. They wait for a long time and adoption is usually the last resort. According to Mrs Nomita Chandy of Aashraya, parents should not wait too long, and adoption should be one of the options instead of being the last option. This is because the whole process of fertility treatment and investigations is not only too traumatic, but also exorbitantly expensive. Adoption can save the couple much of this agony; and often, parents find the process of adoptive parenting so natural that they wonder why they waited so long.

- Some couples adopt out of motives of altruism, in order to give a loving home to a child who needs a home. There are many young couples who want to adopt a second child after having a birth child.

- It is not always for altruistic reasons that parents who have a biological child want to adopt a second one. One of the reasons for adopting a second child is to have a child of the opposite sex. There is no gamble involved in adoption, as there is in the case of having a biological child. Couples might want a boy to continue the family name or to light the funeral pyre.
- Another reason is to avoid the possibility of a known genetic problem that a biological child may have.

Wrong reasons to adopt

According to Mrs Chandy, many people want to adopt a child for the wrong reasons. When the reasons are not right, the adoption agency can turn down the parents because for the agency, the child's rights, privileges and well-being are the top priority. Some of the wrong reasons are:

- Some couples adopt to bring stability to a shaky marriage.
- Adoption is often a way of compensating for a loss or separation, such as the death of another child or divorce. These losses have to be dealt with completely before deciding to adopt.
- A childless mother at home may want to adopt a child because she is bored or depressed.
- Couples should not adopt a child when only one parent wants to adopt.
- Some people adopt because they want a son to perform the last rites.
- Couples may want to adopt because they want a child to take care of them when they grow old or to look after handicapped siblings. Mrs Chandy gave the example of a joint family which belonged to the lower socioeconomic class and lived in a single room. Most of the members had a physical handicap and were invalids, and they wanted to adopt a baby boy who would later look after his elderly parents and handicapped siblings. This was unfair to the adopted

child; their request was turned down.

- Sometimes single people who are younger than 25 years of age want to adopt because they have fire in their belly and want to prove something. They can often be quite impulsive about wanting to adopt when they are single. They also adopt on the rebound, to tide over some sorrow or loss.

According to Mrs Chandy, if Sushmita Sen had approached them for adoption, they would probably have turned her down, for she would not be able to give her child the kind of time that may be required and the child would in reality be brought up by someone else. However, in retrospect, it could turn out to be the best thing that has happened to the mother and child!

It is not the best thing to adopt as a last resort after everything else has failed. It is especially unwise if the parents have not dealt with childlessness per se and accepted it as the reality, because the adopted child will be a constant reminder of their inability to produce a biological child, which is no less than a stigma in our society.

In adopting a baby, the parents' attitude should be one of whole-hearted acceptance and conviction.

The best reason would be: 'I love children and I want to add another member to our family. I want to be a parent.'

This brings us to a fundamental question: Is adoption the second-best option for building a family? Are ties of blood superior in some way to ties of love? To quote an adoptive mother, 'Love transcends many barriers and alters our misguided thinking that true maternal bonding happens only through the umbilical cord.'

Let us now move on to the nitty-gritty of adoption. The next section discusses who is eligible for adoption and what the fears of parents who want to adopt are.

Who can adopt

The criteria for prospective adoptive parents are as follows. (For more details refer to the Central Adoption Resource Agency (CARA) website.[40])

- According to the CARA, the minimum income of those who want to adopt should be Rs 3000 per month. However, Aashraya feels that it should be at least Rs 10,000 to make sure that the child goes into a family that is better placed than the one he/she came from.
- According to the CARA, the minimum educational qualification of the breadwinner should be the Secondary School Leaving Certificate (SSLC) and according to Aashraya, graduation, for the same reasons as above.
- The age of the parents should not exceed 45 years. Older parents can only adopt older children of 3–5 years of age, as it takes a lot of energy to bring up infants and toddlers. Sometimes, older parents do not seem to understand this.
- Younger parents in their thirties can adopt infants or children up to 3 years of age.
- Single parents (male or female) over 30 years of age and younger than 45 are also eligible to adopt. They should have a good support system and a steady source of income.
- Parents who want to adopt a second child can only adopt a child of the opposite sex. If they want to adopt a child of the same sex, the second child will come under the Guardianship and Wards Act and will not be entitled to the family property unless a will is made out.

Many foreigners adopt older children from India and other countries for the following reasons:

- Unwed mothers (the main reason for relinquishing babies in India is due to the stigma of being unwed) are accepted in western countries. Abortion is also more widespread. Hence, there are not many babies available for adoption in the western countries.
- Indian parents prefer infants and as Indian parents are given the first preference, infants are not available to foreigners. That is

the reason why many foreigners adopt older children, as well as children with special needs.

There is a big difference between the number of families wanting to adopt and the number of children available for adoption, especially normal healthy babies, with the former far outnumbering the latter.

Apprehensions regarding adoption

Parents often take a long time to consider adoption as an option for parenting due to various fears. These fears could be about:

- The social and religious background of the child
- Illegitimacy of the child
- Hereditary and environmental influences on the child
- The process of child selection
- Acceptance of the child by the family, friends and neighbours
- Confidentiality of the process
- The possibility of the birth parents trying to reclaim the child.

On birth parents reclaiming child

Agencies want parents to know that the birth parents are given a period of three months in which to change their minds about relinquishment of their child. Once that period is crossed and the child has been adopted, the process is irrevocable in a court of law. So, parents need not really fear that someone will come reclaiming their child. Also, complete confidentiality is maintained in the process and no one can find out where the child has been placed. However, if the birth parents want to know about the welfare of their child, they will be given information on how he/she is doing and are even shown the child's photographs, but no information on the whereabouts of the child is given.

On the other hand, parents who have once adopted a child cannot relinquish that child. For this reason, agencies conduct a detailed home study and counselling; this helps them find out how keen or ready the parents are to adopt. Adoption agencies suggest adopting babies who are 5 months of age or above so that parents do not relinquish a child. Any developmental difficulties are obvious by this time. There have been unfortunate cases in which parents have adopted a newborn illegally from a hospital and have realized later on that the child has special needs. They are not prepared to deal with this and thus want to relinquish the child. Agencies work very hard to avoid such problems and inform the parents about everything they do know about the child.

On open adoption

According to the website *http://www.openadoptioninsight.org,*[41] the primary prerequisite for a truly open adoption is that *the adopted child has the chance of developing a one-to-one relationship with his or her birth family.* Open adoption is not about the adoptive parents bestowing the birth parents with the privilege of contact, nor is it about birth parents merely being available to provide information over the years. Direct contact, in the form of letters, phone calls and visits between the birth family and the adopted child, as well as the adoptive family is essential if they are to establish their own relationships. After all, how can we honestly call an adoption open if the child is not involved?

For many who are just beginning the adoption process, the concept of open adoption appears to be another complication they would rather not deal with. One prospective adoptive mother, weary from years of infertility, asked me at an adoption conference, 'I am pursuing an international adoption because I don't want to have to deal with my child's birth family in any way. What can you say to me that would make me change my mind and pursue, instead, an open adoption?' My answer to her was simply this: 'No matter where your child is adopted from, you will, as adoptive parents, need to "deal with" your child's birth family, whether you know the birth family or not. This birth family is a part of who your child is. Open adoption allows you to know your child better by knowing his birth family.'

Expectant parents considering placing a child for adoption are often just as wary of the prospect of open adoption. Many are told, or feel, that the ongoing contact will make it difficult to move on with their lives. Some are afraid that seeing their child will be too painful. Many worry that their involvement might confuse the child.

Many birth parents in the midst of the crisis of planning for an adoption look upon continuing contact as an option too painful to contemplate. Many adoptive parents, on the other hand, just want to be a family, without the added complication of visits from their child's birth family.

Patricia Martinez Dorner, author of *Children of Open Adoption* and *Talking to Your Child about Adoption*,[42,43] encourages us to see open adoption as just another form of blended family. In adopting, adoptive parents are welcoming the member of one family into their own. This 'blending' of families is not without its share of uncomfortable moments, but the beauty of the birth parents and adoptive parents accepting each other as family is twofold.

One, the birth parents and adoptive parents really get to know each other. It allows them to see who the others are outside of their adoption experience. Being able to know each other as complete human beings allows for greater acceptance. The adopted child is also able to know his birth parents as they are, rather than creating fantasy birth parents.

Two, it gives the child a sense of wholeness. An adopted child whose birth family and adoptive family come together in a familial way will grow up with greater certainty.

Heredity and environment

For parents who decide to adopt, the background of the child is a cause for apprehension. A complete medical examination is arranged and as much information as possible on the birth parents, the pregnancy and delivery details, including the Apgar score (an indicator of the health of a newborn), is collected and given to the prospective parents. Several tests for various illnesses are also conducted.

While heredity provides the potential, it is the environment in which the child grows that moulds and maximizes this potential. Physical characteristics, such as skin, hair, eyes and physical structure, as also attributes such as intellectual potential and talent in music and dance, are determined by heredity. On the other hand, behaviour patterns, personality traits (to a great extent), and mannerisms are all 'acquired' through the process of socialization, identification and role-modelling.

The provision of a nurturing and stimulating environment, along with maximum opportunities for development, facilitates both the physical and personality development of the child. Even a child who is brought up in a neglected, unloved and emotionally deprived environment will blossom in a happy home. He will adopt the adoptive parents' expressions, gestures and behavioural patterns to such an extent that they will often hear strangers remarking that their child resembles them! Most people cannot even guess that the child is adopted until they are informed about it.

It is important for adoptive parents to know about the role of heredity and environment, for people often fear that if the child's father was a pickpocket, he will also turn out to be one. In fact, children adopted by caring parents, who take the time to teach them good values and set good examples by their own behaviour, blossom into productive and contributing individuals. This is well illustrated in the Hindi film *Parvarish*, in which children of a thief and a policeman get swapped. The outcome depends on good 'parvarish' or nurturing that a child gets from his parents—birth or adoptive.

All parents need to have realistic expectations from their children, whether biological or adopted. Adoptive parents who are not well informed about this may tend to blame the birth parents when their children fail to come up to their expectations in order to absolve themselves of their responsibility in the upbringing of their child.

How to 'tell' a child that he is adopted?

Informing the child that he is adopted depends on how comfortable the parents are about the adoption. At Aashraya, a little less than 50% of the parents attend get-togethers for adoptive parents and their children.[44] The rest of the parents do not want their children or anyone else to know of their child's adoptive status.

Why is it important for children to know about it?

The parents will be unable to enjoy their child if they are under the constant stress that he might come to know of his adoptive status from some other source. Family happiness and security cannot be built on an untruth and the fear of discovery. If the child does get to know from an outside source, it will be difficult for him to trust his parents since they had kept such a big secret from him. Therefore, it is advisable to tell the child either when he asks or on one's own. If he does not ask, the parents should initiate a discussion on the subject and share the fact of adoption with him.

What is the right age to tell the child?

According to Mrs Shanti, no age is too early to tell the child about it. The child should be told in a gradual, casual, age-appropriate manner. The issue will keep coming up at various stages and the parents will have to rethink the way they present it according to the age of the child.

How to disclose it?

Usually, parents say, 'I could not have you from my own tummy, so you had to come from someone else's tummy. But you were born for us and we're your own parents forever.' Sushmita Sen is said to have told her daughter, Renee, that 'most babies come from mummies' tummies, but you have come from my heart.'

The best opportunity is when they ask, 'Where do babies come from?' or when someone close to you is having a baby. One can say that not all babies come from the tummy, but some children, like you, also come from a special place where parents look for beautiful babies to take home. One just has to find that magical moment in parenting when children are the most receptive and there is nothing in between—just you and your child.

Parents are advised to take their children to get-togethers for adoptive parents and their children and talk about the matter in a casual and comfortable way. Adoption can be presented as just another way to have babies. To be able to disclose the fact in an appropriate and natural manner, parents themselves must be comfortable with the idea.

Some parents I know have told their children that they will be visiting the very special place where they had first found each other.

Aashraya, where this author used to work (in Bengaluru), hosts regular get-togethers at which adoptive parents and adopted children interact with the children still living in the adoption agency.

Other important issues

There are other issues, such as the child wanting to know about why he was given up. He may also want to find out who his birth parents were.

It is natural for children to want to know why they were given up. I cite here the example of an 8-year-old child who asked her adoptive mother why her birth mother had given her up. She asked, 'Did she not love me?' Her mother replied, 'I don't think that is the reason. How can anyone not love you? You are so adorable. There must have been some other reason.' The mother waited for her daughter to come up with another reason. Then the daughter said, 'Maybe she was too poor to take care of me, so she wanted me to go to a better home.' Such thinking is quite astonishing coming from an 8-year-old.

As for children wanting to know about their birth parents, agencies do not mind giving details without giving the whereabouts. In the USA, agencies follow the practice of open adoption, whereby there is open communication and contact between the golden triangle of birth parents, adoptive parents and children. When Indian children see their American counterparts sharing an open relationship with their birth parents, they too feel the need to find out about theirs. They come to India looking for parents and answers. However, in India, it is legally impossible to disclose the parents' identities. The rationale behind this is that the mothers may be married with children and their own families, and may not want evidence from their past disrupting their peace and harmony. They may not even have disclosed the correct address lest someone tries to trace them. Therefore, meeting one's birth parents is hardly a possibility in India unless the laws are changed.

However, there are many touching stories about adopted youngsters going in search of their mothers and in some cases even succeeding. Often they just want to know why they had to give them up. Once they are able to bring closure to that, they are able to move on in life. Such agony and distress can be avoided in cases of open adoption.

Conclusion

According to Nilima Mehta, the author of *Ours by Choice*, 'In a sense, adoption is both a beginning and an ending; it is the beginning of a lifelong relationship for the couple who have chosen to be adoptive parents; at the same time, for the birth parents, it is an ending—a relinquishment of their parental rights and responsibilities. Both these sets of individuals are facing crises and going through deeply emotional experiences. Yet, the most important individual is the vulnerable child…the focus of all our attention and concern.'[45]

Quoting Judy Rader, an adoptive parent, 'Perhaps an adoptive parent faces sooner what every parent must face eventually: Our children are not ours; they belong to themselves. What will keep them visiting us joyfully when they are grown is the quality of our relationship, not biology. And so it comes to me with a soothing simplicity: I should trust my bond with my daughter. To adopt means "to take as one's own". If I can love another woman's child as my own, why would I think it might be different for my child?'

'"Your daughter looks just like you", someone I know stops me in the street to say. "Thank you", I answer', says Ritu, an adoptive mother.

{ Chapter 12 }

Loss and Grief

And can it be that in a world so full and busy the loss of one creature makes a void so wide and deep that nothing but the width and depth of eternity can fill it up!

—CHARLES DICKENS (1812–1870)

Only people who are capable of loving strongly can also suffer great sorrow, but this same necessity of loving serves to counteract their grief and heals them.

—LEO TOLSTOY (1828–1910)

Sudhir was referred to us for academic underachievement. But that was only a symptom of the underlying problem, which was a perpetual conflict between the parents. He would often end up being the scapegoat when they wanted to get at each other. Eventually, the parents separated, but the child loved his mother dearly and hoped she would come back. When she did not, he was devastated.

Children come across many situations of loss, separation and grief in their young and tender lives. Some of the situations in which they may face loss are:

- when a parent dies or goes away
- when the parents separate or the family breaks up
- the loss of a friend or friendship
- the loss of a pet
- having a disability
- loss of memories due to fire or flood
- the loss of one's culture and homeland when moving to a new country

- the death of a grandparent
- moving house or changing schools
- long periods of separation from a parent
- being in hospital.

Sometimes, children grieve for something that seems small to adults but is big for children, e.g. losing their comforter. Parents who have tried to wean their child off from his favourite security blanket will know exactly what that means.

Children and grief

Growing up is an ongoing process of change that involves losses as well as gains. Changes such as starting childcare or school, sleeping over at a friend's house, changing classes and teachers, or losing a pet, a friend or a family member all bring new challenges and new learning. Depending on the support they receive and how these early losses are dealt with, children can learn to manage and deal with the losses that will confront them later on in life.

Children do grieve, but not in the same way that adults do, and grieving can start at an early age. Children are likely to show their grief in less direct ways than adults. They move in and out of grief. One day they will seem to be fine and another day they will not seem to manage so well.

Children often have more needs at times of loss. This can lead to demanding behaviour as they try to get closeness, care, information, reassurance and support from adults. The experience of loss affects each child differently. The child's age and emotional maturity, the circumstances of the loss and the 'connectedness' with the person or whatever the child has lost are the key factors. It is important to look at each child individually and work out what will best help that child.

A child's experience of grief varies depending on the type of loss and the developmental stage of the child. Moving to a new town may precipitate a grief response that is mild and transient, while grief resulting from the loss of a parent threatens the very foundation of the child's world. Young children express grief in vastly different ways from teenagers and adults.

How children show their grief

Young children, especially, do not have the words to express their feelings the way that adults do. They may not even really know what they feel. Some of their manifestations of grief are:

- suffering from physical pain, such as stomach aches or headaches
- suffering from sleeping problems and getting bad dreams
- suffering from eating problems, such as eating too much or too little
- being destructive
- acting like a younger child
- indulging in angry play or playing the same thing over and over
- not being able to concentrate for long
- developing problems with school work
- being easily upset
- being 'mean' to others
- 'switching off', acting as if they have not taken in what has happened
- acting more like an adult
- showing fear
- showing anger or aggression towards friends, parents or toys
- throwing temper tantrums
- being unhappy and blaming themselves
- showing a tendency to think that the person who has gone was perfect
- crying and giggling without any obvious reason
- displaying clinginess, wanting to be near adults
- running away, avoiding school, stealing
- asking the same questions again and again

- displaying explosive behaviour and acting out.[46]

According to Bruce Perry, the pain of loss is related to the nature of the transition. When loss is sudden and unexpected, there is much less time for the child to begin adjusting. The anticipated death, separation, or move is easier because there has been time to think, anticipate, mourn, and slowly reshape relationships. Gradual, predictable transitions, though painful, make loss easier to deal with.

The pain from loss is also related to the nature of the relationship. A child experiences the maximum distress when he is close to and dependent upon the one he is separated from. If the move or the separation takes the child away from the loved one, he may experience the same intensity of pain as he would have if it were a death.

Stages of grief

'Grief is a process, not a state', according to Anne Grant (1755–1838). For all the traumatic events that we will be talking about, the stages of grief are more or less the same. These stages are generally recognized to be denial, anger or resentment, bargaining, depression, and finally, acceptance. With children the order can vary.

According to Bruce Perry, grief is a process that reshapes our inner world following loss. It involves a set of emotional, cognitive, behavioural and physical reactions that can vary, depending upon the individual and the nature of the loss. During the grieving process, there are two central challenges for the child: (i) Processing the actual event ('What is cancer?' 'Can you catch it too?') and (ii) coping with the loss of the loved one ('I want Daddy to take me to school'). In the weeks immediately following the loss, the child often experiences disturbing thoughts. The primary emotion during this time is fear—fear of the unknown, fear of the future. Over time, the child's thoughts will be dominated by loss and feelings of sadness.

We shall now look at the various losses that children face when confronted with the following:

- Cancer
- Amputation
- Parental separation/divorce
- Death of a parent
- Disasters

Cancer

This is one of those illnesses which is associated with extreme fear, both for the affected person and his family, as it is perceived to be life-threatening. However, great strides in finding a cure have been made in the field of medicine depending on the stage at which it is detected.

Telling your child

One of the most difficult decisions facing parents when their child (or a parent) is diagnosed with cancer is what to tell the child. It is impossible to keep from the child the knowledge that he is seriously ill, because his environment has already told him that he is. The question, then, is not whether to talk about the diagnosis, but rather, how to let the child know that his concerns are shared and understood, and that one is willing to talk to him about these things.

The single most important thing is gentle, honest communication, which should be the basic approach. Failure to answer the child's question in an honest manner undermines the parent–child relationship at a time when the child desperately needs to communicate with his parents. As a parent, one is the best judge of one's child's moods. It must be kept in mind that just because the child does not talk about the illness and the fears related to it (including death), one cannot assume that he does not have these fears.

A child who knows that the illness is more serious than the usual childhood illnesses is undoubtedly afraid. Secrecy tends to isolate him and increase his fears. Exactly when to tell the child and what

CASE STUDIES

When Teja was about five years old, he pleaded with his granny to allow him to buy a few colourful little chickens which were being sold on the roadside. He was allowed to buy just one. He bought it and kept it carefully in a shoe box. He fed it grains and took good care of it. One day, when he was not at home, his friend went over and played with the chicken. By accident, the little chick had a fatal fall from the dining table. When Teja came home and saw what had happened, he was devastated. He was so upset that he did not eat a morsel for three days. He was stricken with grief.

Tara was a little girl of six who enjoyed school and loved her friends. The time had come to send her to a bigger school. When she was finally told that she would be going to a new school and would be making new friends, she took it rather badly. She would throw tantrums, lose her temper and cry, and gave her parents a rough time. She was finding it difficult to cope with separation from her friends and her favourite teacher of three years. But when she did start her journey in her new school, she adjusted very quickly, surprising her parents and herself.

to tell him will depend on his age and maturity, and your attitude. You may prefer to tell the child yourself, whether in the presence or absence of the physician, or you may want the doctor to do it. Use the method that makes you feel the most comfortable.

Age-related concerns

Your physician or other members of the treatment team may be able to help you determine what and how to tell the child. This partly depends on the child's age.

- *Toddlers:* In general, toddlers need only be told that they are sick, that they have to take medicine to get better and that needles hurt, but only for a minute.
- *Under 5:* Separation, abandonment and loneliness are especially frightening to children under the age of 5 years. They need to be reassured that even if they have to leave for a while, they will be back.
- *Between 6 and 10:* Children between the ages of 6 and 10 years, and perhaps as young as 5, have fears relating to physical injury and bodily harm. They understand that theirs is no ordinary illness; it is very serious and threatening. Thus, they need to know that they have cancer, a serious but treatable disease. They may also be told that the cause of cancer is unknown, that they will require many medicines, and that it may take some time before they really feel well again. Much can be said with honesty and hope.
- *Older children and adolescents:* Older children and adolescents are old enough to understand their diagnosis and treatment and also, the implications. They may equate cancer with dying. They need to know not only about their diagnosis and treatment, but also that cancer can often be treated successfully, and about the advances in treatment and increase in survival rates. To these young people, the impact that cancer and its treatment will have on their normal activities, appearance and relationships with their peers may be especially important.

Reassuring your child

Be prepared to cope with questions about death, even if they are painful. Refusing to discuss death may deny your child an outlet for some strong and possibly frightening feelings, and it will deny you the opportunity to offer comfort and reassurance. In addition to discussing the child's feelings and fears, it is important to stress on all young people with cancer the fact that cancer can be treated, that research for better methods is ongoing and that treatments are improving all the time.

Joint discussions between the young person, parents and medical personnel frequently have a soothing effect. The child seems happier knowing about the disease than remaining in fear of the unknown. Medical care becomes more successful because the child can actively participate. Parents do not carry the extra burden of concealing the truth. Despite the uncertainties and the heartaches, everyone becomes more comfortable with the disease and about the future. In addition to talking with their parents and caregivers, young people with cancer may want to read about cancer and hospitalization.

Help your child lead as normal a life as possible. Do not treat him specially or differently, and resist wanting to overprotect him.[47]

Amputation

Amputee management is never a simple situation. It involves much time and effort on the part of not only the patient, but also the family, friends and the healthcare team. When the amputee is a child, the case becomes more complex. Amputation is a mutilation of an individual's body image and produces a sense of finality. It is difficult for many families to accept and understand why their young, innocent child must live life as an amputee. Also, though the parents love their child, they may be unable to cope with his or her limitations.

Developing a positive body image

Child amputees must develop a positive body image and self-esteem to achieve self-acceptance. Body image encompasses physical, psychological and social aspects, and is formed by constantly changing emotions and body perceptions. Disturbances of one's body image occur when changes are not accepted or when previous images do not coincide with reality. If an amputee cannot acknowledge the reality of a missing limb, then he or she may never completely accept his or her body or situation. A child amputee's perception of his or her behaviour and social and athletic ability also significantly affect his or her self-esteem. In addition, extreme emotions and family conflicts may hinder the child's acceptance of amputation.

Generally, support from classmates, parents, teachers and friends, as well as strong family organization and family cohesion, enhance self-esteem and psychological and social adaptation.

Divorce or separation

From toddlers to teenagers, most children of divorced parents feel some degree of blame when their parents end their marriage. They may think that if they had been better behaved, kept their rooms cleaner, studied harder or obeyed their parents more, their parents might have stayed together.

Along with the stages of grief mentioned above, a child may experience many other associated emotions as well, such as sadness, shock, a sense of abandonment or rejection, and shame. Helping your child cope with and understand these expected stages (feelings) can pave the way for positive growth through these experiences, and can lead to cooperation, adaptation, hope and understanding.

Your child may demand more attention—positive or negative—perhaps to test whether you will abandon or reject him. These needs and reactions should diminish as your child adapts to, and accepts, the changes in your lives.

How to help your child cope

Helping your child feel secure and loved will calm him. It will allow him to trust you and to conquer his fear of losing you.

Show your child that you can be trusted. Be there on time to pick him up from school or activities, especially visitations. Do not make promises you cannot keep. Make sure your child knows where and how to reach you by telephone, mobile phone or email.

Maintain a dependable structure

- Keep up the household routines and schedules so that your child will know what to expect. This builds confidence and comforts the child.
- Be consistent with respect to rules and responsibilities, as well as in the way that you respond to the child.
- Work out your daily schedule in such a way that you have adequate free time and flexibility to be able to give your child undivided attention every day.

Understand your child's desire for the other parent

- Whenever possible, allow your child to freely contact the other parent, talk about him/her, and keep his/her photos in his room.
- Encourage your child to write to, call or email the other parent.
- Speak positively to your child about the other parent. Do not expect your child to take sides, spy, or otherwise feel caught in the middle of you and the other parent.

Make visitation a positive, pleasant time

- Be ready at pick-up and drop-off times. Allow your child to take the toys, videos and books he wishes to have with him. Pack appropriate clothing.
- Be cordial to the other parent; do not use this time to discuss issues in front of your child.
- Be flexible when changes must be made to the schedule. Understand that emergencies or unexpected events do take place occasionally.
- Do not withhold visitation without due/legal reasons.

Make your child's life better

- Make sure your child feels confident of himself.
- Spend time together having fun. Take time to enter your child's world and give yourself wholly to him.
- Ask for your child's opinions and ideas on small and big family decisions.
- Praise your child for doing well and trying hard. Let him hear you compliment him to others.
- Be very careful not to criticize or demean your child or the other parent.
- Show your love in every way you can. Give your child plenty of physical and emotional attention.

These steps will help you improve your child's self-esteem, behavioural habits and coping abilities as he goes through the grief cycle.

Red flags for more serious problems

If after several months things get worse rather than better, it may be a sign that your child is stuck in depression, anxiety or anger, and could use some additional support. Watch for these warning signs of divorce-related depression or anxiety:

- Sleep problems
- Poor concentration
- Trouble at school
- Drug or alcohol abuse
- Self-injury or eating disorders
- Frequent angry or violent outbursts
- Withdrawal from loved ones
- Refusal of loved activities.

Discuss these or other divorce-related warning signs with your child's doctor and teachers, or consult a child therapist for guidance on coping with specific problems.[48]

Death of a parent

Developmental phases in understanding death

It is important to recognize that each child has his own unique understanding of death and dying. This understanding depends on the child's developmental level, cognitive skills, personality characteristics, religious or spiritual beliefs, previous experiences with death, the teachings he has received from his parents and significant others and inputs from the media. Nonetheless, there are some general considerations that are helpful in understanding how children and adolescents experience and deal with death:

- *Infants and toddlers:* Very young children may perceive that adults are sad, but have no real understanding of the meaning or significance of death.
- *Pre-schoolers:* Young children may deny death as a formal event and may see it as reversible. They may interpret death as a separation, not a permanent condition. Pre-school children and even children in early elementary school may exhibit magical thinking and link certain events with death. For instance, as a result of the World Trade Centre disaster, some children may imagine that going into tall buildings can cause someone's death.
- *Early elementary school:* Children at this age (approximately 5–9 years) start to comprehend the finality of death. They begin to understand that certain circumstances may result in death. They can see that if large planes crash into buildings, people in the planes and buildings will be killed. At this age, children perceive of death as something that happens to others, not to oneself or one's family.
- *Middle school:* Children at this level have the cognitive understanding to comprehend death as a final event that results in

the cessation of all bodily functions. They may experience a variety of feelings and emotions. Acting out and self-injurious behaviour are among their means of coping with their anger, vengeance and despair.

- *High school:* Most teenagers fully grasp the meaning of death in circumstances such as an automobile accident, illness and even the World Trade Centre disaster. They may seek out friends and family for comfort, or they may withdraw into themselves to deal with their grief. Teenagers (as well as some younger children) with a history of depression, suicidal behaviour and chemical dependency are particularly prone to prolonged and serious grief reactions, and may need careful attention at home and school during this difficult time.

Waldorf schools adopt an interesting and spiritual approach to death, whereby they help the children to start looking at death as something that occurs naturally to everyone and also as a step to something that comes after. Right from kindergarten, through the birthday stories that they are told, they are taught that death is not something bad and that the place we go to after death is like a happy home to which we return and Earth is a place which we have come to just visit and learn. Children are easily able to grasp and accept this due to the magical thinking that they naturally possess at this age.

There is no need for young children to be told hard scientific facts. They will surely learn of these when they are ready for it.

Disasters

Disasters can take many forms. They may be weather-related, e.g. tornadoes, hurricanes or floods; accident-related, e.g. bus or automobile accidents or drowning; illness-related, e.g. arising from AIDS or cancer; or bizarre and unusual, e.g. due to snipers or a murder.

The emotional effects of a disaster on parents and their children can be tremendous. One of the difficulties experienced by parents during disasters is that they have not had adequate time to deal with their own reactions when they are called upon to deal with the impact of the disaster on their child.

Reactions to disaster

Emotional reactions vary in nature and severity from child to child. Children's reactions to a disaster are determined by their previous experiences, their temperament and personality, and the immediacy of the disaster to their own lives. Nonetheless, some commonalities exist between how all children (and adults) feel when their lives are disrupted by a disaster.

Loss of control: By their very nature, disasters are something over which we have no control; if we did, we would stop them from occurring. This feeling of loss of control can be overwhelming.

Loss of stability: Disasters also interrupt the natural order of things. There is a loss of stability and this is threatening; it can destroy trust and upset a person's equilibrium for extended periods. The person is likely to feel that after all, if this disaster could take place, then almost anything else might happen too.

Self-centred reactions: Children's immediate reaction to disaster often includes fear for their own safety. They may be intensely worried about what will happen to them, to an extent that one may consider unreasonable. Young children have difficulty putting the needs of others before their own. Children need repeated reassurance regarding their own safety and the outcome of the disaster, as it relates to them.

Helping children cope with loss and grief

The following tips will help teachers, parents and other caregivers support children who have experienced the loss of parents, friends or loved ones:

- *Allow the child to talk about his grief experiences:* Give the child the opportunity to tell his story. Be a good listener.
- *Make room for individual variations:* Do not assume that every child in a certain age group understands death in the same way or with the same feelings.
- *Grieving is a process, not an event:* Parents and schools need to allow the child adequate time to grieve in the manner that works for him. Pressing the child to resume his 'normal' activities without giving him the chance to deal with his emotional pain may give rise to additional problems or negative reactions.
- *Do not lie or tell half-truths about the tragic event:* Children are often bright and sensitive. They will see through false information and wonder why you do not trust them with the truth. Lies do not help the child through the healing process or help develop effective coping strategies for life's future tragedies and losses.
- *Help all children, regardless of age, to understand loss and death:* Give the child information at the level that he/she can understand.
- *Encourage children to ask questions about loss and death:* Adults need to be less anxious about not knowing all the answers. Treat questions with respect and show a willingness to help the child find his own answers.
- *Do not assume that children always grieve in an orderly or predictable way:* We all grieve in different ways and there is no one 'correct' way for people to move through the grieving process.
- *Let children know that you really want to understand what they are feeling or what they need:* Sometimes children are upset but they cannot tell you what will be helpful. Giving them the time and encouragement to share their feelings with you may enable them to sort out their feelings.
- *Children need long-lasting support:* This is especially true if the child has lost a parent who was his major source of support. Try to develop multiple supports for children who suffer significant losses.

- *Keep in mind that working on grief is hard:* It is hard work for adults and hard for children as well to go through the process of grief and to try and bring it to a closure. Sometimes it may be better to seek help in doing this.
- *Understand that the grieving process is complicated:* Grieving may be complicated by a need for vengeance or justice and by the lack of resolution of the current situation. The sudden or violent nature of the death, or the fact that some individuals may be considered missing rather than dead, can further complicate the grieving process.
- *Be aware of your own need to grieve:* Focusing on the children in one's care is important, but not at the expense of one's own emotional needs. Adults who have lost a loved one will be far better equipped to help children work through their grief if they get help themselves. For some families, it may be important to seek family grief-counselling, as well as individual sources of support.

Professional help

A child who has undergone a trauma needs professional help if he:

- talks of not wanting to live or being better off dead
- seems to be preoccupied with dying
- is unable to concentrate and is withdrawn at school for months after the event
- is crying, sad or depressed much of the time
- does not want to join other children or play with them for months after the event.

Be alert for pathological long-term reactions, which are more severe than those experienced by most children. These might include:

- persistent re-experiencing of the traumatic event through intense recollections, dreams, flashbacks or hallucinations
- persistent avoidance of stimuli associated with the trauma or

numbing of responsiveness—restricted affect and diminished interest in the usual activities
- signs of increased arousal, such as sleep difficulties, irritability, hypervigilance, disturbances in concentration, or exaggerated responses.

Conclusion

Children are not very good at putting their feelings in words. Their agony is often expressed through behaviour which the adult world mostly judges negatively, blaming the child for his behaviour. Little help is available for such children in terms of counselling and intervention. When they are on the way down, they are often labelled as cases of attention deficit disorder (ADD) or attention deficit hyperactivity disorder (ADHD), or as 'slow learners' or 'troublemakers', and when they go down too deep, they may need to be criminalized, hospitalized or even buried.

If we could just see them in a new way, we could help them better. Together, as a support team, we could learn to really see them and hear them, we could learn the signs and recognize their pleas for help before they turn into screams, and before the screams are forever silenced.

{ Chapter 13 }

Sexuality Education

Let's begin this topic with an interesting anecdote. A mother had given her 12-year-old son a Childcraft book which had information on reproduction, and he read about sperm and eggs. A few days later, he saw his cousin with her newborn baby (apparently he had not attended her wedding). In surprise, he asked her, 'How did you get a baby?' She was amused and asked him, in turn, 'What do you think?' Without any delay, he replied (to the shock of all those around him), 'Oh! All you need is sperm and eggs!' This illustrates the adage, 'knowledge is power', but half-baked knowledge can be dangerous when it comes to sexuality.

What is the one word that comes to one's mind at the mention of sexuality? The following have been the responses of a few people who were asked this question:

- 'Sex'
- 'Sex appeal'
- 'Sexual organs'
- 'Sexual expression'
- 'Sex education for young children'
- 'Power' (control over oneself, and that translating into power and freedom)
- 'Passion'
- 'Intimacy'
- 'Aggression'
- 'Gender discrimination'
- 'Depicting your inner self', because ultimately that is what matters.

These responses indicate that sexuality is not just about sex. It is about knowing who you are, being comfortable with who you are, your identity, rights, roles, the right to correct information, preventive education, values, decision-making, assertiveness, conflict resolution, safety, and so on.

When does it begin?

When does the aspect of sexuality begin? Is it during puberty, or is it during pre-puberty? The fact is that it begins much earlier. Sexuality education is something people think of only in the context of adolescents and teenagers. However, the aspect of sexuality starts before birth. This does not mean that the baby is a sexual being, thinking sexual thoughts. To begin with, the sex of the child will influence the attitudes of the parents towards him/her, his/her identity, parental expectations and attitudes, and so on. The aspect of sexuality comes into play in the following ways:

- When the parents discuss whether they would like to have a boy or girl, and their reaction when the child is born
- When the parents debate on whether to get their baby pink clothes or blue clothes
- Whether the parents get all worked up on seeing their baby playing with or exploring his/her genitals, and how they react
- Whether the parents give the child a doll or a car to play with
- Whether they allow their son to cry, or whether they say, 'Boys don't cry!'
- Whether they encourage their little girl to be a tomboy.

Thus, the whole gamut of sexuality begins very early on. Sexuality is not just about sex education and the age at which it should begin. It is also about attitudes, beliefs, values and the comfort levels of the parents, teachers and significant others in dealing with various issues related to sexuality.

Parents' ideas on sexuality

Often, the topic of sexuality gives rise to a sense of uneasiness among people. Parents think teachers should enlighten their children, while teachers think it is the parent's job. Perhaps the discomfort arises because we are not sure what to think. What are our values? Are they realistic? Are our beliefs realistic? Do we just silently pray that our children will be fine and that nothing will happen to them? Or do we believe that today's youngsters are very smart and do not need to be taught? Or do we even believe that by talking about it, we may actually be implanting ideas where there were none?

Before parents attempt to give their child education on sexuality, it may be worthwhile for them to sit together and examine what their values are. What do they want their children to know? Do they agree or can they decide to agree on what they think is important for their child to know? Who will do the talking?

Checking whether you agree or disagree with the following statements will help you find out how comfortable you are with sexuality and what your beliefs about sexuality-related issues are.

- Boys and girls should have the same toys in their toy chests.
- Infants should be allowed to touch their genitals.
- I would not mind if my child is homosexual when he/she grows up.
- It is the mother's job to teach the child about sexuality.
- Children need to know the correct names of their genitals.
- It may not be wise to teach the child about sex too early.
- I want to be the one to teach my children about intercourse.
- Parents should closely monitor what children watch on television.
- Parents should set the dress standards for their children until high school.
- I want my child to wait until marriage to have sexual intercourse.

Some sexuality-related issues

We shall now address some of the major sexuality-related issues that confront parents and attempt to find answers to the most common of these.

Answering children's questions: There is a mistaken notion that education on sexuality should begin just before puberty or even in adolescence. This is in spite of the fact that parents commonly come across various situations much earlier, in which their children ask them sexuality-related questions, which they do not know how to answer. Sex education is not a one-time activity or a question of giving one's child some basic information, then heaving a sigh of relief and thinking, 'Ah! I've done it. I've managed to answer the dreaded question!' Children are not satisfied with this. Even as one is answering a question, the next one is already taking shape. They will surely come back with the next missile; one has to be prepared. The nature of their questions will change as they grow. Sex education is a continuous process which begins when the child starts asking questions. It is better if it is we who answer the questions, and that too truthfully, rather than the child getting incorrect information from unreliable sources.

Tips to deal with sexuality-related questions

Debra Haffner, the author of *From diapers to dating—A parent's guide to raising sexually healthy children,*[49] gives us the following advice.

- *Do not just wait for the questions:* Some children are brimming with questions, but some never ask. Do we wait for our children to ask how to cross the road? We do not. Sexuality is as important as matters like how to cross the road and it is our job as parents to give our children the right values. One has to decide what is important about sexuality for the children to know, and then find time and ways to tell them.
- *Reward your children's questions:* Tell your children you are glad that they asked so that they will be encouraged to ask again. Make sure you mentally prepare yourself to be able to answer them. If you realize the importance of doing this, you may not feel so embarrassed when faced with their questions.

CASE STUDY

Simmi (age 5, jumping on the bed): 'Girls drink Pepsi to become sexy.'
Mom (surprised but acting casual): 'Where did you hear this Simmi?'
Simmi: 'On the bus! All the girls say it!'
Mom: 'What does sexy mean?'
Simmi (still jumping on the bed): 'Sexy means strong. I drink Pepsi, so I am strong mama!'
Pammi (age 15, whispering): 'Maa! Change the topic!!'

- *It is all right if you do not know the answer:* It is also all right if you do not know how to answer. If you do not know the answer, say so. You can tell the child that you will find out the answer and get back to him, or you can find out together. If you do not know how to answer, ask for some time and say that you are not ready. However, in both cases, get back with an answer, letting your child know that you can be believed.
- *It is all right if you are uncomfortable:* If you are not comfortable answering a particular question (especially personal questions about your relationships), feel free to say so and tell the child that if he wants to know more about relationships in general, you will be glad to talk about it. As for general questions that you are uncomfortable with, you could take your child to someone who can answer them for you, like a gynaecologist or a doctor. But tell your child that you do want to talk to him about these issues because you love him.
- *Educate both your sons and daughters:* Parents, especially mothers, are more comfortable educating their daughters than sons. However, education is important for both. A woman can ask her husband to help and she can help him by preparing together.

- *Practise if you want:* Some parents find it useful to rehearse in front of the mirror to feel comfortable before they do the actual talking.
- *Find 'teachable' moments:* Sexuality educators define 'teachable moments' as the times that arise naturally when information on sexuality can be provided easily. Some examples are when you are watching television together, reading the newspaper or listening to the radio in the car, or when you find your child in a sexual situation. You can identify such situations and take advantage of them to impart the right values regarding sexuality.

  According to one parent, her job has been made easier by the television channel 'Animal Planet', through which her daughter has learnt about the process of natural childbirth in mammals. The girl asked her mother if she, too, was born that way, and her mother seized the teachable moment to explain the difference between natural birth and a caesarean section. She also learnt that a male and a female are required to mate and to produce offspring. The girl was matter of fact about it and there was no look of embarrassment on her face. To her, this was just another piece of information in the lifelong process of learning. It is only we who feel embarrassed. Sometimes we transmit this embarrassment, as well as negative attitudes and concepts (such as sex is dirty or disgusting) to our children through our tone of voice, demeanour and facial expressions, thus passing on faulty notions about sex.
- *Use words and ideas that are appropriate for your child's level of development:* Find out how much the child knows before you jump in with your input. When your son asks you where he came from, you may launch into an explanation of all the biological details, and your son may say, 'But my classmate says he has come from Hyderabad!'

  Parents also fear that too much information may harm the child. However, there is no need to worry because research shows that learning about sex does not cause children to experiment. Pamela Wilson, a sexuality educator, tells parents to give the simplest possible information and give more details only if the child asks for them.

- *It is all right to make a mistake:* If due to your own lack of awareness you have given faulty information to your child, or if you have handled a situation inappropriately, you can make up for it. It is all right to say that you are sorry and that you were wrong. In fact, it teaches the child that no one, not even mum or dad, is perfect.
- *It is never too late to start:* Although education on sexuality begins in infancy with the kinds of messages we convey through our own actions, it is never too late to start sexuality education. No matter what age your child is, he just needs to be given truthful, age-appropriate information.

Child sexuality is different from adult sexuality

Parents often find their children playing with their own genitals or exploring those of their friends. This shocks and perplexes them and they feel unsure about how to handle it. First of all, parents need to realize that child sexuality is different from adult sexuality. Parents get anxious because they look at children's behaviour from an adult point of view. But, all that the child is exhibiting is a naive and natural curiosity to find out about his own and others' bodies. It is necessary for parents to know how to react, as their reaction will influence the child's attitude towards sex when he grows up. Parents should try hard to remain calm and ask what game the child is playing. They should make sure that the child does not get the opportunity to be left alone for at least a few days. There should be absolutely no shouting or scolding. The parent can tell the child that no one has a right to touch one's genitals except oneself.

Child playing with his/her own genitals and masturbation

If your child is 2–5 years old and you find him playing with his genital area, gently distract him with some other activity. By this, you are conveying that it is not bad to masturbate. If a child is constantly stimulating himself, it could signify some stress, insecurity or even abuse. You may need to find out more about what is happening in your child's life.

When you find that your older child, irrespective of whether or not he has attained puberty, is masturbating, do not be shocked or alarmed. You may have done it yourself, but must have felt guilty or ashamed about having done it. There is nothing shameful about masturbation. It is a natural biological need for both males and females, although the need is greater among males. It fulfils some important needs, such as relieving sexual tension, providing a safe means of sexual experimentation, controlling sexual impulses and discharging general stress. If the child is masturbating excessively, try to find out if something is troubling him.

Preparing them for puberty

Children will have many doubts, fears and anxieties about their changing bodies. But they may not feel like asking anyone about these things. It is important that in this phase of one's child's life, one should bring up the topic oneself rather than wait to be asked. The child may never ask. Girls need to be told about menstruation before puberty. They must be told why and how it happens, and should also be instructed about the aspect of hygiene. Boys need to know why new things are happening to them and should be assured that these are perfectly normal. Both boys and girls need to be reassured about their growth, and it is important to address any concerns or complexes they may have about their size.

Safety and protection

Teenagers are not only precocious, but also experimentative. They are under pressure to conform. Children at this age have a very strong need to feel accepted. Exposure to issues related to sexuality is much higher than earlier, thanks to the media and internet, and sometimes children are exposed to material for which they are biologically not even ready.

This kind of exposure may stir certain feelings in the child, increasing his curiosity. This has made sex education about safety and protection against date rape, unwanted teenage pregnancy and of course, AIDS and other sexually transmitted diseases not only important, but also necessary and urgent.

Girls are attaining menarche earlier than ever and the average age for marriage is increasing. At the same time, the average age for starting pre-marital sex among girls in India is dropping.

A large-scale survey was conducted in 2010 under the aegis of the Union Health Ministry in the six states of Andhra Pradesh, Bihar, Jharkhand, Maharashtra, Rajasthan and Tamil Nadu. The results came as a shock for those opposing the introduction of sex education in Indian schools. Pre-marital sex has been found to be common among young men, and the percentage of women between ages of 15 and 24 years who have had sex before reaching the age of 15 has risen.[50]

Child sexual abuse

Children need to be taught about safety, not to talk to strangers, not accept sweets from strangers and about 'good touch' and 'bad touch'. This has to be done not in a serious or grave manner, but casually as an opportunity comes up naturally. This is to ensure that children do not needlessly develop new fears but know about safety issues if and when the need arises, and are able to voice their concerns.

Signs of sexual abuse

Does your child

- Have nightmares, sleep too little or too much?
- Have an extreme fear of the dark or 'monsters'?

- Have a loss of appetite or trouble eating or swallowing?
- Have sudden mood swings: rage, anger, fear or withdrawal?
- Fear a certain person or place? (A child may not want to be left alone with a babysitter, friend, relative or other child or adult.)
- Complain frequently of stomach illness with no identifiable reason?
- Engage in sexual activities with toys or other children, such as simulating sex with dolls or asking other children to behave sexually?
- Use new words for private body parts?
- Refuse to talk about a 'secret' he has with an older child or adult?
- Talk about a new older friend?
- Suddenly have money?
- Cut, burn or harm himself or herself as an adolescent?

Other signs include excessive masturbation, excessive crying, wearing many layers of clothing and vaginal discharge or bleeding.

In the case of any of the above, consider taking the child to a specialist to rule out the possibility of sexual abuse.

The most important aspect of rehabilitation is to convince the child that the abuse is not her fault and that she is in no way responsible for what has happened.

One child, a teenager admitted to a hospital, was so traumatized after being sexually abused that she had no memory of what happened after the traumatic event. She was happy to be in the in-patient department and talk about everything but the event.

Children and homosexuality

While hostility to homosexuality was well established in western society for centuries, an important shift in attitudes occurred around 1900. Some physicians and other sex researchers began to claim that people were either homosexual or not. The idea that people could have a combination of both homosexual and heterosexual interests, which had been a common experience for some groups, was increasingly downplayed in favour of the new dichotomy. Further, homosexuality was now regarded by many as a disease, rather than simply a form of immorality. With this new approach, and with the growing emphasis on the importance of heterosexual dating and other activities for older children, concerns about signs of homosexuality among children increased. Parents and children themselves became increasingly anxious about homosexuality, and it became a major element of child-rearing and socialization after the 1920s. While the most recent developments have loosened the strictures on homosexuality, elements of this earlier tradition persist as well.

In the twentieth century, more data became available and the study of childhood sexuality became systematized, although studies are very difficult to do except retrospectively, that is, through people's reported memories of their own childhood activities. We know that children learn early on what sex they are. In most cultures a child is easily identified as a boy or girl by the clothes he/she wears and what his/her parents and others tell him/her. In fact, usually the first question asked about a newborn is what sex it is. Though children gain a gender identity some time between one and two years of age, they do not yet have a sense of gender constancy. A little boy may believe, for example, that at some later point in life he will be a girl. Even though the overwhelming majority of children soon realize this is an error, many keep wishing they were of the opposite sex and try to act like they are, and this seems to be a strong disposing factor for later transsexualism and homosexuality. Children's unwillingness to accept their assigned gender roles is often very difficult for parents and other adults to accept.[51]

Attitudes toward homosexuality are very personal and differ from family to family. The attitudes of children towards homosexuality or the guilt they experience when they are attracted towards people of the same sex will depend on the attitude of the parents.

Moreover, gay or not, they are people first. Why should anybody's identity as a human being be reduced to their sexual orientation?

With new laws creating space for LGBT (lesbian, gay, bisexual, and transgender) individuals in the world, there is now increasing acceptance of gay relationships. This reminds me of the way a friend used to joke about her son: 'I do not care whom he marries as long as it is a girl.' People may be willing to accept LGBTs in general, but when it comes to their own child, there is an underlying fear of one's child being gay.

Sexuality and special needs

Sexual development is a multidimensional process, intimately linked to the basic human needs of being liked and accepted, displaying and receiving affection, feeling valued and attractive, and sharing thoughts and feelings. It not only involves anatomical and physiological functioning, but also relates to sexual knowledge, beliefs, attitudes and values. Sexuality should be considered in a context that extends beyond genital sex to include gender-role socialization, physical maturation and body image, social relationships, and future social aspirations. Like all adolescents, teenagers with disabilities may express the desire to marry, have children and lead normal adult sex lives. In fact, adolescents with physical disabilities are as sexually experienced as their peers without disabilities. However, parents and healthcare professionals are often pessimistic regarding the potential of children with disabilities to enjoy intimacy and sexuality in their relationships. People with disabilities are often erroneously regarded as childlike, asexual and in need of protection. Conversely, they may be viewed as inappropriately sexual or as having uncontrollable urges. People without disabilities are more willing to accept people with disabilities as fellow employees or casual friends and less willing to accept them as dating, sexual or marriage partners. Societal and psychosocial barriers may be more of a hindrance to an adolescent's sexual development than the limitations of the disability itself.

Historically, sterilization of minors with developmental disabilities was performed without appropriate regard for their decision-making capacities, ability to care for children, feelings or interests. Such decisions should be made only in the context of the individual's capacity to make decisions, the consequences of reproduction for the person and any children that might be born, and applicable local, state and federal laws.

It is important to encourage the development of self-esteem in children with disabilities. Like all children, those with disabilities feel better about themselves and are more readily accepted by their peers when provided with smart and age-appropriate clothing that is easily donned. Social development is largely experiential, and children with disabilities generally have fewer opportunities for social interactions than their typically developing peers. Promoting typical teen activities, such as going to the mall or a movie with peers or participating in social activities at school, may require extra parental planning, but afford invaluable opportunities to develop social skills. By mastering appropriate greetings, eye contact, body language, issues of personal space, self-advocacy skills, and telephone and computer skills, children build a strong foundation for the development of more complex social skills.

Children with disabilities may be more vulnerable to sexual abuse because of their dependence on others for intimate care, increased exposure to a large number of caregivers and settings, inappropriate social skills, poor judgement, inability to seek help or report abuse, and lack of strategies to defend themselves against abuse.[52] These fears may lead parents to protect their children from unsupervised social contacts and even from knowledge of sex. Some fear that talking about sexuality will promote sexual behaviour. Yet, lack of education poses greater risks. When sexual questions and the behaviour of individuals are freely discussed within a family, sexual development is promoted and the likelihood of abuse may be reduced or eliminated.[53] Children can learn to be assertive in protecting the privacy of their own bodies and in reporting violations to trusted adults.

Children with disabilities have the right to the same education about sexuality as their peers, but often the programme must be modified to allow the information to be presented in such a way that the child can understand and learn it. The modifications that may be required include simplifying information, teaching in a special needs setting rather than a regular education setting, using special teaching materials such as anatomically correct dolls and teaching methods such as role playing, and frequently reviewing and reinforcing the material. Individualized education plans (IEPs) should include the provision of sexuality education for children with disabilities. An appropriate programme for children with disabilities includes the following topics: Body parts, pubertal changes, personal care and hygiene, medical examinations, social skills, sexual expression, contraception strategies, and the rights and responsibilities related to sexual behaviour.

This goal of providing sexuality education for individuals needing special care is best accomplished when parents are the principal teachers and offer sexuality education appropriate to the cognitive and functional abilities of their child.

Sexual precocity

Words like 'sexy' are being used most casually in the media, including on the front pages of newspapers and popular songs that children sing. 'Munni' and 'Sheela' have become household names. Newspapers carry sensational pictures and celebrity gossip that sometimes border on porn. The standards have come down and people are accepting them as normal. The reality shows today are playing a major role in encouraging children to act like adults. We see them performing suggestive dance movements, with competitive parents egging them on. Some parents do not think twice about dressing up their daughters in revealing outfits, buying them their own make-up and even taking them to the beauty parlours for waxing and threading at a tender age, when they should be playing innocent games.

Schools can play an important role in sexuality education in the following ways:

- They can impart education on sexuality, but this will be useful only as far as giving facts is concerned.
- Probably a better thing to do would be to find out from the students themselves what they would like to know.
- Schools need to conduct life skills education courses, through which children are taught skills such as decision-making, conflict resolution, assertiveness training and self-esteem to prepare and empower them for the numerous challenges they will be facing in their lives. Gender, family values, relationships and responsibilities, and sexuality should all be covered in these courses.
- As part of the curriculum, teachers can be trained to look out for 'teachable moments' in classes like English, languages and science. The teacher can find out how much the children know and what their opinions are on various issues related to gender and sexuality, and can also encourage healthy debates on various points of view. For this to be successful, however, teachers, as in the case of parents, need to have a certain level of comfort and an idea about their own beliefs on sexuality-related issues.

Children are losing their innocence earlier than ever due to over-exposure through television and the internet. We find children talking about 'going steady', and 'boy/girl friends' at increasingly younger ages. Their minds are maturing faster than their bodies. How far can parents try to protect their children from getting information?

The only way to protect children is by giving them the right values and education. It is not enough to give our children facts. One of the most important jobs of any parent is to make sure that his/her children have their values in place. The child may have many thoughts and temptations, many opportunities to try out new experiences. But acting on them is an entirely different matter. Some of the life skills issues that only parents can empower their children to deal with relate to questions like, 'How far can I go about fulfilling my desires? Where do I draw the line? When and how do I say no? Why do I need to respect another person's privacy?'

In a survey in which students were asked what changes could lead to a better understanding of sex, the students responded that their parents and teachers needed classes in sex education before imparting it to their children.

Conclusion

Sexuality education is the process of assisting young people in their physical, social, emotional and moral development as they prepare for adulthood, marriage, parenthood and ageing, as well as their social relationships in the context of family and society. The need to impart appropriate education on sexuality is an important issue that parents and teachers must acknowledge and address if they want to make sure that their children are well adjusted and safe, and will grow up to be mature and balanced individuals.

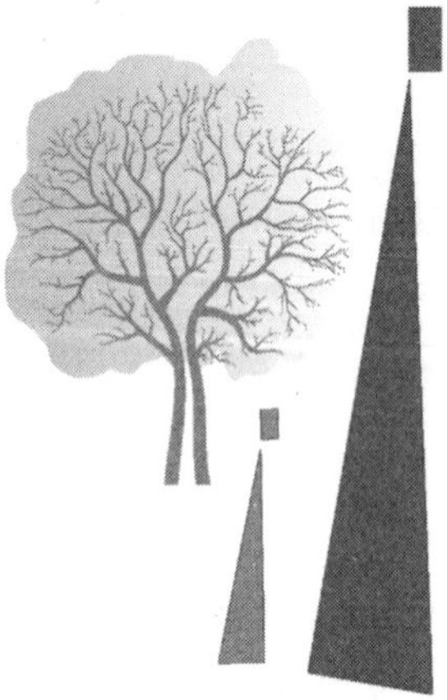

Glossary

(ANTHROPOSOPHICAL) CURATIVE EDUCATION. Curative education and social therapy have their origins in the early 1920s and the pioneering work of the Austrian philosopher and educator, Rudolf Steiner. Curative education is an interdisciplinary approach to addressing the unique needs of people with developmental disabilities. It involves the integrated use of practices taken from remedial pedagogy, medicine and psychiatry, a variety of therapeutic techniques, and from the arts. These practices are tuned to the developmental needs of each individual; in fact, the specific challenges and potential of each person are the starting point for all curative education work.

Curative education is based on the understanding that the student and teacher are closely interdependent, with each contributing to the other's psychological and spiritual development.

ANTHROPOSOPHY. This is a spiritual philosophy, developed mainly by Rudolf Steiner (1861–1925) at the end of the 19th and beginning of the 20th century. While rooted in a philosophy of freedom and an impulse to nurture a purely human interest in other people, and developed as a method of spiritual research, it also has possible practical implications. Applied or practical anthroposophy forms the basis of various 'daughter movements' of anthroposophy. These include Waldorf education, anthroposophic medication, biodynamic agriculture, anthroposophic architecture, eurythmy and curative education (special education).

ASPERGER SYNDROME. This is a mental condition similar to autism. It is a condition that makes it difficult for someone to react to and communicate with other people. It is similar to autism, but less severe.

ASPHYXIATION. When a person or animal is deprived of oxygen, usually leading to unconsciousness or death, it is known as asphyxiation.

AT RISK. A person is at risk when he/she is exposed to a potentially risky circumstance which increases the probability of a compromised developmental condition, such as premature birth, delayed birth cry and low birth weight.

ATTENTION DEFICIT HYPERACTIVITY DISORDER (ADHD). This is a group of behavioural symptoms that include inattentiveness, hyperactivity and impulsiveness. The common symptoms of ADHD include a short attention span, restlessness, being easily distracted and constant fidgeting. Many people with ADHD also have additional problems, such as sleep disorders or learning difficulties. However, ADHD has no effect on intelligence.

ATTENTION DEFICIT DISORDER (ADD). This is a type of attention disorder where the distractions are more internal, where the child cannot concentrate due to inadequate filtering mechanisms of the stimuli coming in from the environment.

AUTISM SPECTRUM DISORDER (ASD). This is a neurobiological condition in which the use of language, reaction to stimuli, interpretation of the world and ability to form relationships are not fully established and follow unusual patterns, causing a disturbance in psychological development.

EPILEPSY. Epilepsy is a medical disorder involving episodes of irregular electrical discharge in the brain and characterized by the periodic sudden loss or impairment of consciousness, often accompanied by convulsions.

EXPRESSIVE LANGUAGE DISORDER. This is a communication disorder in which a person has difficulty with verbal and written expression. It is a specific language impairment in which the ability to use expressive spoken language is markedly below the appropriate level for the mental age, but language comprehension is within normal limits. There can be problems with vocabulary, producing complex sentences and remembering words, and there may or may not be abnormalities in articulation.

Care must be taken to distinguish expressive language disorder from other communication disorders, sensory–motor disturbances, intellectual disability and/or environmental deprivation (*see* DSM-IV-TR criterion D). These factors affect a person's speech and writing to certain predictable extents, and with certain differences.

FERAL. This describes animals or plants that live or grow in the wild after having been domestically reared or cultivated.

INTELLECTUAL DISABILITY. This term is used in the case of a person who has certain limitations in mental functioning and in skills such as communicating, taking care of himself or herself and social skills. A child with these limitations will learn and develop more slowly than a typical child.

Children with intellectual disabilities (sometimes called cognitive disabilities or mental retardation) may take longer to learn to speak, walk and take care of their personal needs, such as dressing or eating. They are likely to have trouble learning in school. They will learn, but it will take them longer. There may be some things they cannot learn.

LEARNING DISABILITIES. These conditions either prevent or significantly hinder a person from learning basic skills or information at the same rate as most people of the same age and intellectual level.

PERVASIVE DEVELOPMENTAL DISORDER–NOT OTHERWISE SPECIFIED (PDD-NOS). This is one of the autism spectrum disorders and is used to describe individuals who do not fully meet the criteria for autistic disorder or Asperger syndrome.

PDD-NOS may be thought of as 'subthreshold autism', or a

diagnosis one can give a person who has 'atypical symptomatology'. In other words, when someone has autistic characteristics but some of his/her symptoms are mild, or he/she has symptoms in one area (like social deficits), but none in another key area (such as restricted, repetitive behaviour), he/she may be given the PDD-NOS label.

SCHIZOPHRENIA. This is a severe psychiatric disorder characterized by symptoms of emotional instability, detachment from reality and withdrawal into the self.

SEMANTIC PRAGMATIC DISORDER (SPD). This is a language disorder first defined by Rapin and Allen in 1983. It describes children who present with mild autistic features and specific semantic pragmatic language and communication impairments. SPD is separated into two groups: Receptive and expressive language. SPD is characterized mainly by poor conversational skills with inappropriate use of language, and receptive language becomes difficult because comprehension of words is unclear.

SYNAPSE. The small junction across which a nerve impulse passes from one nerve cell to another nerve cell, a muscle cell or a gland cell. The synapse consists of the synaptic terminal, or presynaptic ending, of a sending neuron, a post-synaptic ending of the receiving cell that contains receptor sites, and the space between them (the synaptic cleft).

SYNAPTIC PRUNING. In neuroscience, synaptic pruning, neuron pruning or neuro-structural re-assembly is a neurological regulatory process which facilitates a productive change in neural structure by reducing the overall number of overproduced or 'weak' neurons into more efficient synaptic configurations. It is often used as a synonym to describe the maturation of behaviour and cognitive intelligence, through the 'weeding out' of the weaker synapses, in children.

SYNDROME. A syndrome is a group of signs and symptoms that together are characteristic or indicative of a specific disease or other disorder.

THE MONTESSORI METHOD. This method of bringing up and educating children aims to see children as they really are and to create environments which foster the fulfilment of their highest potential—spiritual, emotional, physical and intellectual—as members of a family, the world community and the cosmos.

TRANSACTIONAL ANALYSIS (TA). Eric Berne designed TA as a system that seeks to understand the interactions of people and to improve the human social environment. Almost 50 years after the inception of TA and 30 years after the untimely death of Eric Berne, it has become a movement with thousands of members all around the world. It is poised to enter the third millennium as a highly effective, information-based approach to the psychology of human communication.

WALDORF EDUCATION. Developed by Rudolf Steiner in 1919, Waldorf education is based on a profound understanding of human development that addresses the needs of the growing child. Waldorf teachers strive to transform education into an art that educates the whole child—the heart and the hands, as well as the head.

References

Chapter 1

1. MacLean K. The impact of institutionalization on child development. *Dev Psychopathol* 2003 (Fall);**15:**853–84. [kmaclean@stfx.ca]
2. Prescott JW. Grand Rounds. *Behavioral mismanagement of newborns: Impact of social isolation and sensory deprivation.* Childrens Hospital. National Medical Center, 9 September 1976.
3. Itard, Jean-Marc-Gaspard. *The wild boy of Aveyron.* New York: Meredith; 1962.
4. Rymer, Russ. Annals of science. I-*A silent childhood.* New York; 1992:41.
5. Prescott JW. Rock A Bye Baby. (30 minutes). Time–Life Films. New York; 1970. [http://www.violence.de/tv/rockabye.html]

Chapter 2

6. http://www.childdevelopmentinfo.com/development/normaldevelopment.shtml

Chapter 3

7. http://psychology.about.com/od/developmentalpsychology/a/parenting-style.htm
8. Maccoby EE, Martin JA. Socialization in the context of the family: Parent–child interaction. In: Mussen PH (ed) and Hetherington EM (Vol. ed). *Handbook of child psychology: Vol. 4. Socialization, personality, and social development.* 4th ed. New York: Wiley; 1983:1–101.
9. Coloroso, Barbara. *Kids are worth it!* Toranto, Canada: Penguin; 2001.
10. Steiner, Rudolf. *Education in the light of anthroposophy*; 1965.
11. Steiner, Rudolf. *The Four Temperaments: Lecture in Berlin.* (ISBN 0910142114). http://wn.rsarchive.org/Lectures/FourTemp0s/ForTem_index.html;1909.
12. Amy Chua. *Battle hymn of the tiger mother.* (ISBN 9781594202841).

Chapter 4

13. http://www.learning-theories.com/piagets-stage-theory-of-cognitive-development.html

14. Gardner, Howard. *Frames of mind: The theory of multiple intelligences.* New York; 1983.

Chapter 5

15. Pelzer, Dave. *A child called "It".* Health Communications Inc., Deerfield Beach, Australia.
16. Bretherton, Inge. The origin of Attachment theory: John Bowlby and Mary Ainsworth. *Developmental Psychology* 1992;**28:**759–75. http://www.psychology.sunysb.edu/attachment/online/inge_origins.pdf
17. Sharma, Robin. *Family wisdom from the monk who sold his Ferrari.* Mumbai: Jaico.
18. Faber Adele, Mazlish Elaine. *How to talk so kids will listen and listen so kids will talk.* Collins; 1999.

Chapter 6

19. Soanes C, Stevenson A (ed). *Generation gap.* The Concise Oxford English dictionary. [Online]. Oxford: Oxford University Press. Oxford Reference Online. BLC Boston College Libraries. Retrieved June 8, 2005 from http://www.oxfordreference.com/views/ENTRY.html?subview=|Main&entry=t23.e22836.
20. Barker RL. (2003). *The social work dictionary* (5th ed). Washington, DC: NASW Press; 2004:176.
21. http://www.therebelution.com/blog/2007/10/study-shows-teens-love-family/
22. 'Kushboo enlarged on bail'. *The Hindu* 2005-11-17. http://www.hindu.com/2005/11/17/stories/2005111720110100.htm

Chapter 7

23. Vera Rabie-Azoory. Sibling rivalry: The truth about the family favorite. WebMD Live's Family Wellness Auditorium.
24. Faber Adele, Mazlish Elaine. Siblings without rivalry. Copyright© 1987, 1998 by Adele Faber and Elaine Mazlish. Summarized by permission of the publisher, HarperCollins Publishers. ISBN: 978-0380799008; ISBN10: 0380799006. Summary Copyright ©2010 by FamilyIntel, LLC. All rights reserved.
25. Faber Adele, Mazlish Elaine. *How to talk so kids will listen and listen so kids will talk.*

Chapter 8

26. *Atkinson & Hilgard's Introduction to Psychology* (15e) (ISBN-13: 9781844807284).
27. Smith MK. *Learning theory.* The encyclopedia of informal education; 1999. www.infed.org/biblio/b-learn.htm, Last update: 03 September 2009.
28. Ramsden P. *Learning to teach in higher education.* London: Routledge; 1992:4.
29. Ramsden P. *Learning to teach in higher education.* London: Routledge; 1992:26.
30. http://us1.campaign-archive1.com/?u=a0ce04e5a70babb8ef1330163&id=d4b2aa20d2&e=22e5d262bf
31. Miller J. 2005. http://innovativelearning.com/teaching/social_learning_theory.html
32. Orr 2005. http://seli.stanford.edu/research/documents/aera_07/orr_learning-leadership_matters.pdf
33. http://newglobaled.org/(the quotes of Nancy Meaker, J. Krishnamurthy and Dalai Lama have been sourced from this site).
34. Steiner, Rudolf. *An introduction to Waldorf Education* (1919). The Anthroposophic Press; 1985.

Chapter 9

35. Berne, Eric. *Games people play.* New York: Grove Press; 1964. ISBN 0-14-002768-8.
36. Pelzer, David J. *A child called "it": One child's courage to survive.* Omaha; 1993.

Chapter 10

37. http://www.waldorfhomeschoolers.com/teaching-family-values
38. Dubey, Scharada. *The best days of my life.* Scholastic; 2010.
39. Koehler, Michael D. *Football coach's survival guide.* Parker; 1992.

Chapter 11

40. http://adoptionindia.nic.in/index.htm
41. http://www.openadoptioninsight.org/what_is_open_adoption.htm
42. Talking to your child about adoption. Tree of Life Publishing; 1991.
43. Silber Kathleen, Martinez Patricia. *Children of open adoption.* Dorner: Corona; 1990.

44. http://www.nriol.com/ashraya
45. Nilima Mehta. *Ours by choice*. Mumbai: Rite-Print-Pak; 1992.

Chapter 12

46. www.griefspeaks.com
47. http://www.cancer.org/Treatment/ChildrenandCancer/WhenYourChild HasCancer/Children DiagnosedwithCancerDealingwith Diagnosis/index
48. http://www.helpguide.org/mental/children_divorce.htm

Chapter 13

49. Haffner, Debra. *From rdiapers to dating—A parent's guide to raising sexually healthy children.* Magna; 2000.
50. http://zeenews.india.com/news/newspapers/sex-before-15-girls-pip-boys-study-the-times-of-india_605825.html
51. http://www.faqs.org/childhood/Gr-Im/Homosexuality-and-Sexual-Orientation.html
52. http://aappolicy.aappublications.org/cgi/content/full/pediatrics;118 /1/398
53. http://www.childwelfare.gov/pubs/factsheets/signs.cfm

Suggested reading

Chapter 2 – http://fmfeat.tripod.com/indicato.htm
Chapter 3 – http://www.athealth.com/practitioner/ceduc/parentingstyles.html
Chapter 3 – www.theparentingpassageway.com
Chapter 5 – http://0.tqn.com/d/psychology/1/0/-/4/attachment2.jpg
Chapter 9 – http://www.spiritwire.com/selfesteemquotes.html
Chapter 9 – Harris A. Thomas. *I'm ok—you're ok*. Arrow Books.
Chapter 11 – http://www.adoptionopen.com/adoptionquotes.html
Chapter 12 – http://teacher.scholastic.com/professional/bruceperry/death_and_loss.htm

Index